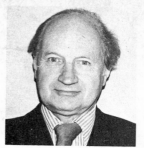

GW00382863

Doctor Anthony C. Turner, comes from a family of four generations of doctors, of which three have been authors of medical and other books. He qualified in 1942 at King's College Hospital where he initially held resident appointments before serving on flying units in the Royal Air Force until the end of World War II. He then spent eleven years in general practice in England and Kenya.

In 1956 he joined British Overseas Airways Corporation as adviser on tropical and overseas medicine and to be responsible for the care of their overseas staff and families. In 1965 the medical departments of B.O.A.C. and B.E.A. merged to become subsequently British Airways Medical Service. The same year he was appointed a visiting lecturer at the London School of Hygiene and Tropical Medicine (Hospital for Tropical Diseases) and in 1975 he became an Honorary Associate Physician at the Hospital for Tropical Diseases.

Retiring from British Airways in 1981 he was appointed a Consultant Medical Adviser to the Civil Aviation Authority and Boeing International Corporation. In 1982 he opened the Medical Advisory and Immunisation Centre at Trailfinders Travel Centre. He is also consultant medical adviser to Travellers Medical service, one of the major medical assistance organisations. For the last twenty years he has been adviser to the British Olympic Association on tropical and travel medicine. He is President of the International Association of Physicians for the Overseas Services. He is consultant editor of the *Journal of Tropical Medicine and Hygiene* and on the editorial board of *Travel Medicine International.* In 1975 he published *Travel Medicine, a Handbook for Practitioners,* and in 1987 *First Aid and Home Safety.* He has written many articles in medical and other journals on the medical problems of travel with particular regard to businessmen, athletes and families. He is a regular contributor to the journal 'The Expatriate' and has appeared frequently on Radio and Television to discuss these problems.

For Daniel and Louisa

THE
TRAVELLER'S
HEALTH
GUIDE

Dr. Anthony C. Turner
Consultant in Tropical and Travel Medicine

By the same author
Travel Medicine, a Handbook for Practitioners
First Aid and Home Safety

Roger Lascelles, Cartographic and Travel Publisher
47 York Road, Brentford, Middlesex TW8 0QP. Tel: 081-847 0935

Publication Data

Title	Traveller's Health Guide
Typeface	Phototypeset in Compugraphic Times
Printing	Kelso Graphics, Kelso, Scotland.
ISBN	0 903909 87 1
Edition	First Jan 1971, Second May 1979, Third Dec 1985, Fourth May 1991.
Publisher	Roger Lascelles
	47 York Road, Brentford, Middlesex, TW8 0QP.
Copyright	Dr Anthony C. Turner

Distribution

Africa:	South Africa —	Faradawn, Box 17161, Hillbrow 2038
Americas:	Canada —	International Travel Maps & Books, P.O. Box 2290, Vancouver BC V6B 3W5
Asia:	India —	English Book Store, 17-L Connaught Circus/P.O. Box 328, New Delhi 110 001
	Singapore —	Graham Brash Pte Ltd., 36-C Prinsep St
Australasia:	Australia —	Rex Publications, 413 Pacific Highway, Artarmon NSW 2064. 428 3566
Europe:	Belgium —	Brussels - Peuples et Continents
	Germany —	Available through major booksellers with good foreign travel sections
	GB/Ireland —	Available through all booksellers with good foreign travel sections
	Italy —	Libreria dell'Automobile, Milano
	Netherlands —	Nilsson & Lamm BV, Weesp
	Denmark —	Copenhagen - Arnold Busck, G.E.C. Gad, Boghallen, G.E.C. Gad
	Finland —	Helsinki — Akateeminen Kirjakauppa
	Norway —	Oslo - Arne Gimnes/J.G. Tanum
	Sweden —	Stockholm/Esselte, Akademi Bokhandel, Fritzes, Hedengrens Gothenburg/Gumperts, Esselte Lund/Gleerupska
	Switzerland —	Basel/Bider: Berne/Atlas; Geneve/Artou; Lausanne/Artou: Zurich/Travel Bookshop

Contents

Appendices

Foreword

(First Edition)

Professor A.W. Woodruff C.M.G., O.B.E.
PhD, FRCP, MD, FRCP(Edin), DTM & H.
Emeritus Wellcome Professor of Clinical Tropical Medicine
of the University of London.

The British Overseas Airways Corporation make a point of the fact that they take good care of their passengers. The attitude which they and their staff adopt is clearly underlined by Dr Turner's book. It is a frank and personal account of the measures he recommends for taking care of the modern traveller's health. He has gone into the whole range of the traveller's health needs with great care and detail. He speaks with very great experience of these needs after years of study of and practice in the ways of maintaining their health. He puts forward his advice in an easily understood and reasonable manner. This book is one which therefore can be recommended with confidence and is bound to fill a greatly felt need.

1

Background

Air travel on the scheduled services of the member airlines of the International Air Transport Association increases by 10 to 15 per cent annually, so that over 950 million people travelled on these services in 1988. This figure does not include all those who went abroad on inclusive tours or charter services or enjoyed sea cruises, so the ultimate figure is far greater; 250 million were on international services.

Not only are people travelling in much greater numbers but also, with the increasing speed of travel, they are going progressively farther afield. Holidays are no longer confined to western Europe and the northern shores of the Mediterranean as they were for the first 15 years after the end of the 1939—1945 war. The eastern and southern shores of the Mediterranean soon became involved and then the Caribbean, South America, East Africa, the Seychelles and the Far East fell to the ever more enterprising holidaymaker. At the present time Thailand is one of the most popular countries, with the development of their beautiful beach resorts, as is Bali for similar reasons. Backpacking is becoming ever more popular, and the overlanding trips through Africa and across Europe and Asia to India and Nepal are booming.

Additionally, business and sales personnel from the United Kingdom have set forth across the world selling their goods and services as successive prime ministers, of whatever political colour, have instructed them. The British technician is still required in many developing countries of the world whether he is employed by a British, American or local company. Most of them travel by air and find themselves suddenly deposited in new climates and environments which present new health problems. Some of the illnesses which develop may be mild, causing only a few days' sickness, though even that can spoil a costly family holiday. On the other hand, a serious illness such as malaria may develop which can kill quickly — in a few days. But malaria, like many other medical problems of foreign countries is preventable.

Even so the incidence of malaria imported into the United Kingdom has increased nearly 20 times over the last 20 years. One hundred cases were notified in 1970, 1,447 cases in 1977 whilst throughout the last decade there have been on average 1,800 cases each year. This is a preventable disease and travellers may not be doing everything possible to protect themselves.

In Chapter Two I shall discuss all the vaccinations and immunisations that travellers should have before going abroad. There are two definite groups:

● those which are required by international regulations;
● those which are not legally essential but are very important for medical reasons.

Whichever and however many are necessary, it is most important for travellers to have them in good time before setting out. If possible at least six weeks should be allowed.

Following pre-travel immunisations, advice is given on how best to enjoy the journey, whether it is by air or sea, and how to be best equipped to cope with the new climate and environment on arrival.

A few simple principles, easily followed, will enable the new arrival to cope quickly with the tropical heat. Diseases of the tropics and semi-tropics can be divided into three main groups:-

1 Those caused by insanitation
2 Insect-borne
3 Those transmitted by direct contact including bites and stings.

Surveys have shown that around 50 per cent of all travellers, mainly to Europe and the Mediterranean, have suffered from minor ailments such as diarrhoea, colds and sunburn. Accidental injuries are common, in particular pedestrians forgetting that traffic is driven on the right, and minor accidents are frequent around swimming pools and on dirty beaches.

One must remember that "tropical diseases" are not necessarily limited by the Tropics of Cancer and Capricorn. Malaria, for instance, occurs along the North African coast which is so popular with the holidaymaker. In 1969, 38 cases of typhoid were known to have occurred amongst holidaymakers who stayed at the same hotel in Tunisia; in 1984 there was an epidemic in the Greek island of Kos; and in 1989 there was an outbreak on the Costa Dorada in Spain. Around 200 cases of typhoid are diagnosed in the U.K. every year, of which at least 90 per cent are imported.

On the more cheerful side, there has probably been a greater advance in preventive medicine with regard to the tropical diseases than in any other branch of medicine. By following some simple precautionary principles most problems can be avoided.

In Appendix A the question of overseas medical facilities and the cost of medical care abroad is considered. A lot of criticism is levelled at the National Health Service. Some of this criticism must be valid but the general public in the United Kingdom tends to forget how much medical care can cost and also takes a lot for granted. The need to take out an insurance policy is discussed as also are the administrative problems of the E.E.C. countries.

Appendix D lists the climate and vaccination requirements for all countries. Needless to say these are the requirements at the time of going to press. If in doubt you should get in touch with the embassy, consulate or High Commission of the country or countries you are intending to visit.

Those travelling overseas who are on regular medical treatment should be careful to take with them an adequate supply of all necessary medicines, sufficient for their whole stay if this is practical. In addition, all medicines should be very clearly labelled both with the proprietary and the pharmaceutical name. This is necessary because, although the actual medicine may well be available abroad the name may be different. Your pharmacist can help you by putting both names on the bottle label.

Under U.K. National Health Service regulations you are not entitled to obtain any medicines which are for use overseas so you may well have to purchase them privately, but it is an expense well worth accepting. In many places abroad they could cost more.

It is essential that anyone has sufficient medicines for the journey available in their hand luggage and this amount must allow for any delays. One has known of diabetics who have packed their insulin and syringes in their baggage which is unavailable in the aircraft hold. All bottles of liquid medicine should have screw tops and not corks.

Should you fall sick on your return from a visit overseas or shortly afterwards it is essential that you tell your doctor that you have been abroad and where you have been. This will alert the doctor to the fact that your illness may be related to your travel.

If you have had malaria abroad, tell him, because malaria may recur for up to one year or more after you have left the malarious area.

2
Pre-travel immunisations

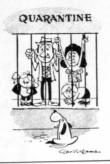

QUARANTINE

With the advent of the World Health Organisation after the 1939—1945 war certain regulations were laid down regarding travellers passing to and through areas of the world where certain severe diseases may occur. Up to 1970 these regulations were known as the International Sanitary Regulations, but at that time the name was changed to the International Health Regulations which is far more appropriate.

All members of the United Nations are automatically members of the World Health Organisation and most of them are signatories of the International Health Regulations. The most notable exceptions are Australia and Singapore, whilst India, Pakistan and Sri Lanka have certain reservations regarding yellow fever.

There were three vaccinations which were covered by these regulations, namely those against smallpox, cholera and yellow fever. Signatories of the International Health Regulations can enforce these requirements by quarantining travellers who are not vaccinated. With the eradication of smallpox there are now only two.

Many people refer to these injections as inoculations reserving the term vaccination for smallpox. Technically this is quite correct although the World Health Organisation likes the term vaccination to be used for all three of these preventive measures. Vaccination is derived from the Latin word *vacca* meaning "cow" because smallpox vaccine is derived from "cowpox". None of the other immunisations has anything to do with the cow. Hence the incongruity of W.H.O. terminology.

There are other inoculations which are advisable for the traveller and which on many occasions are far more necessary for medical reasons but are not required by international law.

Vaccinations covered by International Health Regulations

However for those specifically mentioned above a valid certificate of vaccination must be produced by the travellers under circumstances which shall be described.

Form of certification

This certificate must be on the approved form laid down by the government of the country of issue and in accordance with the International Health Regulations. On no account will a letter from a medical practitioner or a certificate on a medical practitioner's headed notepaper be accepted as valid. In the past, if you were vaccinated by your general practitioner, then you had to take the certificate to the local area health authority to be authenticated with a rubber stamp. Matters have now been simplified and the private practitioner has certificates which he can authenticate.

There are also certain authorised vaccination centres around the country where internationally required vaccinations can be given. Their authentication is sufficient.

Smallpox

The recent history of the complete eradication of smallpox throughout the world is probably the greatest success story of W.H.O. In 1963 smallpox occurred in over fifty countries in the world. Ten years later in 1973 it was present in Pakistan, India, Bangladesh and Ethiopia. By 1977 it was found only in Ethiopia although it had been imported into Somalia and Kenya. It was on 23 October 1977 that Ali Maow Maalem in the township of Merka in Somalia became the last person in the world to be notified as suffering from smallpox. On 1 January 1980 the W.H.O. announced that the world could now be considered free from smallpox. Despite this, it was several years before every country agreed not to demand smallpox vaccination. Up to 1983 it was still demanded by Chad but now, happily, no country demands it.

This success story is so fascinating that a brief history of the origin of vaccination is worth mentioning because it is by world-wide vaccination that smallpox has been eradicated in 180 years.

It was in 1798 that Edward Jenner first published his paper on the benefits of vaccination. In the countryside of Gloucestershire where he lived there had been an established tradition that dairymaids who had contracted cowpox from the cows they milked did not contract smallpox. Cowpox produces blisterlike sores, both on the udder of a cow and on the human skin. These resemble the sores of smallpox, but the disease is very mild. It is not spread from human to human. Early in his medical studies Jenner conceived the idea of applying, on a large scale, this method of preventing smallpox. Later, when he studied at St George's Hospital, London, under the great John Hunter, he told the latter of his idea. Hunter gave him advice which was charactertistic of that great surgeon and investigator. He said, "Don't think, try: be patient, be accurate." Jenner returned to his home, and for 18 years he patiently collected his observations on the protection against smallpox given by cowpox. In 1796 he was willing to try his idea. He performed his first vaccination upon a country boy named James Phipps using matter from the cowpox sores on the arms of milkmaid Sarah Nelmes, who had acquired the cowpox from the animals she milked. Two months later he inoculated the boy with pus from a case of smallpox. The boy did not contract the disease.

Initially Jenner's ideas were rejected by the Royal Society, but in time they were accepted by that august body and as has already been written through the last 180 years vaccination has been established as the one great prophylactic measure against smallpox. And so the names of James Phipps and Sarah Nelmes at the beginning and Ali Maow Maalem at the end can go down in the history in eradication from the world of one of the most appalling diseases.

Cholera

Cholera is an acute infective diarrhoea looked upon as Asiatic in origin, in particular occurring in India, Pakistan and China. However, the El Tor variety has recently spread from South East Asia to the Middle East and in 1970 to Southern Russia through the Balkans and into Saudi Arabia. From the Arabian Peninsula it was introduced into Ethiopia through the port of Djibouti by smugglers crossing the Strait of Bab el Mandeb by dhow and then carrying their goods by camel train. From Ethiopia it spread north, west and south until by 1971 it was found in North Africa and briefly in Spain. Later still it spread from North Africa to Italy and caused a short-lived epidemic in Naples.

By 1970 therefore the travellers need for cholera vaccination had greatly increased. Whereas previously it was necessary for travellers passing through India and Pakistan to the Far East and Australia, it suddenly became necessary too for travellers to the Middle East and Africa.

However, in December 1970 in Washington, the then Surgeon General of the United States Public Health Services, Doctor Jesse

Steinfield, announced that cholera vaccination certificates would no longer be required from travellers coming to the United States from cholera infected areas. Thus the United States became the first country to adopt this official position. He went on to say that there were no doubts about the efficacy of smallpox and yellow fever vaccines, but there was clear evidence that cholera vaccine was of little use in preventing the spread of cholera across borders.

The decision of the United States of America was based on the understanding that whilst the introduction of cholera into a country could not be prevented by vaccination its spread can be prevented only by proper surveillance and containment of diarrhoeal diseases in cholera areas and, most important, improvement of sanitation.

The last severe cholera epidemic in Britain was that known as the Broad Street Pump Epidemic of 1849. Broad Street was in Soho, London and a Dr John Snow was the general practitioner who attended most of the 500 cases which occurred. He wrote a classic description at that time which could hardly be bettered with our modern scientific knowledge. He wrote "Cholera travels along the great tracks of human intercourse never going faster than people travel and generally much more slowly. In extending to a fresh island or continent it always appears first at a seaport. Its exact progress from town to town can not always be traced, but it has never appeared except where there has been ample opportunity for it to be conveyed by human intercourse". He further went on to write of this epidemic that "minute quantities of the dejections of cholera patients must be swallowed and unless these persons are scrupulously clean in their habits and wash their hands before taking food they must accidentally swallow some of the excreta and leave some on the food they handle and prepare". A classic description of a food hygiene problem which should be accepted by all food handlers — and written 130 years ago.

The crux of the matter lies in adequate public health services and adequate sanitation, because in the developed countries cholera does not spread.

At the 26th World Health Assembly in June 1973 it was recommended that vaccination against cholera should no longer be required as a condition of admission to any country. As member states would have to agree and international legal ratification laid down, the 1973 regulations were to continue until at least 1 January 1975. In 1990 several countries still demanded vaccination against cholera certification from travellers entering from countries where there are current outbreaks. At present there are around 7 in these categories compared with 29 in 1985.

It is not necessary to have two injections, as is frequently thought. Validity of the vaccination starts six days after the injection and lasts for only six months. If revaccination occurs within the six months there is no six-day waiting period. In general it is not required for infants under one year but some countries demand it at any age.

For the traveller to countries which demand a valid certificate one intradermal injection of cholera vaccine is sufficient. Canada refuses to give cholera vaccination. Their doctors sign the certificate stating there is no medical indication for it. This may not satisfy a difficult health officer at the point of entry into a country. I have had several Canadians come to my clinic and ask to be given cholera vaccination as, sensibly, they do not want to be given an injection by a local 'health officer'. However for someone who is living where there is a severe outbreak of cholera then it is best to have two subcutaneous injections preferably four weeks apart, but this can be cut to one week if absolutely necessary.

Yellow fever

Yellow fever vaccination is the last mandatory vaccination. It can be considered as one of the greatest advances in modern preventive medicine, in that it has changed a killer disease into a non-runner.

Yellow fever, originally known as yellow-jack, was a scourge of the early explorers and their ships' crews when they visited the American shores from New York down to Rio, and also the equatorial shores of East and West Africa. In 1793, 10 per cent of the population of Philadelphia died of yellow fever. As late as 1865 a few cases were verified in Swansea, South Wales. It was yellow-jack in the 1880's which prevented the French from building a canal across the Isthmus of Panama. So great was the mortality from the disease during their work that it is said there is a Frenchman buried under every tie of the Panama Railway. It was in 1881 in Cuba that it was first suspected that the disease was spread by a mosquito. Dr Carlos Finlay, who was considered to be a theorising old fool, first preached this idea without proof. In 1898—1900 in the Spanish-American war in Cuba, many American troops were dying of yellow fever and the American Government set up a Yellow Fever Commission. It was headed by Major Walter Reed and Dr Finlay's ideas were considered. Volunteers stepped forward to be bitten by mosquitoes which had previously bitten patients dying from yellow fever. Dr Jesse W. Lazear of the Commission died of yellow fever as a result of this, leaving a widow and two children. James Carroll, father of five, also developed a severe attack of yellow fever but somehow survived. To be certain that it was mosquito-borne, three

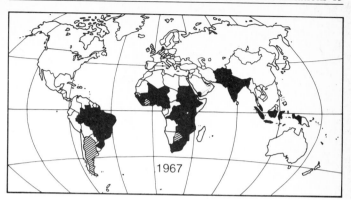

World wide state of smallpox eradication
shaded areas = infected areas
striped areas = imported cases

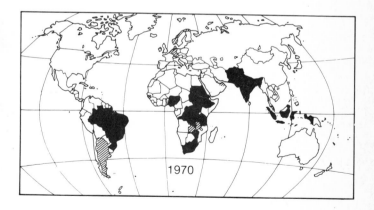

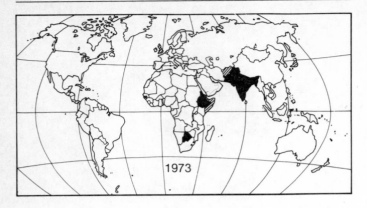

World wide state of smallpox eradication
shaded areas = infected areas
striped areas = imported cases

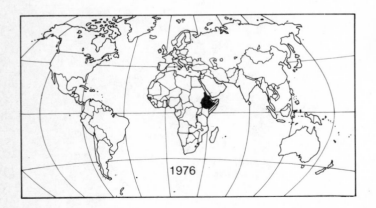

other volunteers — Cooke, Folk, and Jernegan — slept in bed clothes soiled with the black vomit of men who had died of yellow fever, but in mosquito-proofed accommodation. They did not develop yellow fever. From this Reed, Carroll and Agramonte discovered that yellow fever was a virus infection spread by the *Aedes* family of mosquitoes, and mainly the *Aedes Aegypti*. The *Aedes* is a different family of mosquitoes from the *Anopheline* which spreads malaria. Yellow fever vaccination is an absolute guarantee against catching yellow fever.

Immunisation is required only for travellers to Central Africa and Central America: in Africa from 15° north of the Equator to 10° south, and in America from the northern border of Panama state, but excluding the Canal Zone, to 15° south of the Equator, excluding certain areas of Eastern Brazil (see map). In all these areas transit in the international airports does not count as exposures to an endemic area except for travellers arriving in India or Pakistan within six days of transitting these airports. However, all travellers to these areas must be fully protected in their own interest and, although there is officially no lower age limit, most countries do not demand protection of infants under 12 months. There should be an interval of at least 21 days between yellow fever vaccination and any other vaccination with a live virus, except poliomyelitis. Poliomyelitis should be given at the same time or three weeks apart.

The giving of yellow fever vaccination should be avoided during pregnancy and on no account should be given to anyone suffering from Hodgkin's disease, leukaemia or AIDS.

There is a ten-day waiting period after the giving of the vaccine before the certificate is valid, but it lasts for 10 years.

Remember it cannot be given by private practitioners and it is only given in specially-designated centres.

Medically recommended vaccinations

There are other vaccinations which are strongly recommended on medical grounds but are not mandatory. They can all be given to the traveller by his own practitioner and at some of the specially designated centres.

Typhoid

The first is the inoculation against the enteric group of diseases, namely typhoid and paratyphoid A and B. It is generally thought that anyone travelling outside north-western Europe, Canada and the northern states of the U.S.A. should be inoculated against these diseases. It must be remembered that they are particularly common around the Mediterranean littoral. With the inclusive tour holiday boom, resort areas of the Mediterranean are subject to seasonal population explosions. Some of these resorts which are new, only recently developed and with doubtful sewerage services, are potentially endemic areas because of the sudden strain put on the public health services.

In the U.K. there is now only one type of vaccine known as the monovalent typhoid vaccine for these diseases. However, in Europe they produce what we used to know as "T.A.B.", which is a vaccine against typhoid, paratyphoid A and paratyphoid B. It was produced in the U.K. but has recently been discontinued as it was felt not to be very effective against paratyphoid B. In the past there have been personal objections against vaccination against these diseases in that the vaccine can cause a generalised upset for up to 48 hours. However, with modern vaccines this is now far less frequent and with the new technique of injecting the vaccine into the skin for slow absorption, rather than through the skin (subcutaneously), unpleasant symptoms are rare.

A suggested course of monovalent typhoid is to have the second injection four weeks after the first. However, this interval can be decreased to two weeks or increased to eight weeks if necessary. Boosters should be given every three years, but if there is a high risk then every year is advisable.

If time is short before departure one injection is better than none at all. A fair immunity of short duration is provided and should be enough to cover one short holiday although unsatisfactory for the frequent traveller. The course of injections should be completed on returning home after the first trip. It is essential for the camper who is visiting the continent, especially the Mediterranean, to be protected against typhoid, as it is for the overlander.

VIVOTIF, an oral typhoid vaccine, is used in Western Europe, Australia and the U.S.A., but is not available in the U.K. It consists of taking three pills on three different days within one week (total of nine). In the U.S.A. they recommend four capsules. Trials have shown that it is 60 to 70 per cent effective but the monovalent typhoid is considered to have a 70 to 90 per cent effectiveness.
Note In Germany typhoid is called abdominal typhus, when in fact Typhus is a completely different disease — so beware.

Tetanus

Tetanus is far commoner in the developing and warmer countries than it is in the U.K. so every traveller should be protected. Another reason is that if they cut themselves overseas they are less likely to go to a local doctor or hospital because they have no knowledge of them or their whereabouts. And thus they would not receive a post-injury inoculation which is essential unless you have been inoculated in the last 12 months.

For active immunisation against tetanus the initial course is of three injections of the toxoid, the second six weeks after the first and the third six months after the second. Booster doses should be given within 10 years in the U.K. However if someone is at risk after receiving an open wound, particularly if dirty, they should be given a booster dose of toxoid if the last dose was more than a year ago.

Care must be taken to realise the difference between tetanus toxoid (TT) and anti-tetanus serum (A.T.S.). The former, to which we have been referring up to now, gives active immunity and is non-toxic. A.T.S. gives only passive immunity after injury and is short lasting, for the one injury only. The major problem with A.T.S. is that it is developed from horse serum and it can cause severe problems in people who have allergic problems, eczema or asthma. Hence another important reason to have active immunisation with tetanus toxoid. Once someone has had this they need never be subjected to the risk of A.T.S., which, incidentally, is no longer given in the U.K., but is still given in some developing countries. Because of this, it is sensible for the traveller to have a booster every five years.

Poliomyelitis

The third disease to be considered, against which protection is absolutely essential for the traveller, is poliomyelitis. Because of the excellent campaign of poliomyelitis vaccination which has been carried out in countries such as the U.K. over the last 30 to 35 years one tends to forget what a problem it still is in the developing countries.

Poliomyelitis is basically a disease of warm climates, it is spread in the faeces and hence the spread is greater where sanitation is poor. When it strikes in adults it is often more severe. A few years ago Gregory and Spalding, from the Respiratory Unit in Oxford, reported two businessmen who had contracted poliomyelitis whilst on brief business tours to the tropics. They were both over 30 years of age and both are now confined to artificial respirators for the rest of their lives. We may look upon poliomyelitis as a disease of children and young people, as the old name of infantile paralysis infers, but it can strike later in life.

Three drops of the Sabin oral vaccine is the method of choice. The second dose is four to eight weeks after the first and the third a similar time after the second. Boosters should be given every five years. It is of paramount importance for the traveller to have a booster at least every five years. However, it should not be given if there is any diarrhoea present at the time. Pregnant women, if they have to have a course, should be given the Salk vaccine by injection. This vaccine is also used in the presence of an acute epidemic. The oral vaccine should be given three weeks before or after yellow fever vaccination. If this is not possible it must be given at the same time.

Gamma Globulin for Infective Hepatitis A

This is an inoculation which, during the last few years, has been recommended more often and has become far more accepted.

Hepatitis A is an inflamation of the liver in which one of its symptoms is jaundice. It is spread by infected faeces so it is common where food hygiene is poor and water polluted, including water used for swimming as well as drinking. Gamma Globulin should be given whenever it is necessary to immunise against typhoid, i.e. all travel outside north-western Europe, Canada, the U.S.A., Australia and New Zealand. Rumours have been spread that gamma globulin can give you AIDS, it is not effective, and when the injection has worn off you are more likely to develop infective hepatitis. All three points are nonsense. Firstly it cannot give you AIDS or spread AIDS. Although it is a blood product it is heat treated and so any chance of infectivity is killed. Extensive trials have been carried out by the American Peace Corps and the U.K. Voluntary Service Overseas. In each case infective hepatitis was prevented during the period of activity of gamma globulin. After the period of effectiveness the incidence of hepatitis was the same as with a group who had never been given gamma globulin. The smaller dose gives helpful protection for two months and the largest dose for six months. It is an intramuscular injection and can cause local discomfort for a day or two.

Plague

This inoculation is far more frequently recommended in the U.S.A. than in the U.K. The reaction to the inoculation can be very severe both generally and locally. Because of the reaction it must not be given at the same time as typhoid. It is only advisable for upland and mountainous areas of Africa and South America.

Two injections should be given at 10 to 20 day intervals with a third six months later. The validity is six months. Because of its very limited need it is difficult to obtain.

Rabies

With the spread of rabies across Europe the problem of protection against this horrible disease has come even more to the foreground. Once established, rabies is fatal, so everything must be done to prevent this. There have been three fatal cases of rabies in Britain in the last few years: two of the people had been bitten by dogs in India, and one by a dog in West Africa. However, in France there may be over 1,000 cases of animal rabies notified in a year — mainly in foxes.

How then does one prevent this dreadful disease?

● Firstly, by maintaining in the United Kingdom the six months quarantine rule on pets brought into the country. Apart from one case of rabies in a dog in Camberley in 1969, there has not been a case of animal rabies in the U.K., other than in quarantine, since quarantine was started approximately sixty years ago.

● Secondly, elsewhere there must be more vaccinations of all dogs.

● Thirdly, there should be a reduction in the number of wild life animals which spread the disease: in particular wolves and jackals. It is important to remember that in a country where rabies is endemic any animal could be rabid: it is not necessarily confined to foxes, dogs, or cats because any animal could have been bitten by a rabid animal.

● The fourth and most important point is that anyone who has been bitten by a **possibly** rabid animal must receive prompt treatment to prevent the fatal disease developing.

Until recently rabies vaccines were toxic and so prophylactic vaccination was recommended only for veterinarians and those working with veterinarians. However a new vaccine, the diploid tissue cell vaccine, has recently been produced in France. Two doses are given at an interval of four weeks and a third is given 12 months later. A booster should be given every two or three years if exposure continues. Since the vaccine is still in comparatively short supply it is expensive. Treatment in the form of vaccine and serum is still absolutely essential after being bitten or if an open wound has been licked. Immediate first aid is to wash the bite or wound with plenty of water and soap or a detergent. It should not be scrubbed as this can force the infection, if any, further into the blood stream. The vaccine is generally available at the special yellow fever immunisation centres.

Some clinics give a small intradermal dose to make the injection cheaper. However, some authorities think that the protection is not as great when given this way and prefer the standard method. Further, if given intradermally the second injection must be given at least one month before travel and the taking of chloroquine as a malarial preventive also upsets the immune response. Anyway if bitten by a **possibly** rabid animal, you must seek treatment immediately, probably at a major centre. The injections give you extra time to get treatment: they definitely do NOT cut out the need for treatment.

Hepatitis B

Hepatitis B is a more serious but less frequent disease than Hepatitis A. It is spread by direct inoculation with infected blood, either by blood transfusion or transplacentally or through sexual intercourse, and is also spread by clinically dirty needles and syringes. It is estimated that there are over 200 million carriers of Hepatitis B worldwide. In parts of South East Asia approximately 10 per cent of the population may be infected. The following groups of people going overseas must be immunised against Hepatitis B.

● Medical Staff, nurses and laboratory staff
● Those who may need medical or dental treatment to any extent
● Those likely to have several sexual partners

In general it is advisable for all who intend to live in developing countries to be immunised against Hepatitis B. It would be sensible for tourists who are 'backpacking' across South America, Africa and/or Asia for over six months to be immunised. A new vaccine for Hepatitis B, called Engerix B, is effective. The best programme is one dose followed by a second dose one month later and a third dose six months later. If a faster programme is necessary then a third dose can be given after two months and a fourth dose must be given after 12 months. Because of the problems with AIDS and Hepatitis B all expatriates and preferably all tourists should have their blood groups tested before going abroad. Then it may be possible, if a blood transfusion is necessary, to have a colleague, relative or friend to act as a donor. Certain organisations make up emergency medical kits which consist of sterile disposable syringes and needles, sterile suturing packs (stitches), blood-transfusion-giving sets and in larger kits bottles of a blood expander and dextro-saline, to give instead of, or as a temporary measure before, a blood transfusion. Such organisations are M.A.S.T.A. at the London School of Hygiene and Tropical Medicine, British Airways Immunisation Centres and Trailfinders Medical Advisory and Immunisation Centre at 194 Kensington High Street, London, W8.

Meningococcal Meningitis

There are several types of meningitis, an inflammation of the coverings of the brain, which is a serious disease. It can be viral in origin or bacterial, when it is known as meningococcal meningitis. There are several types of the bacterial type, known as A,B, and C. There is a new vaccine against A and C. Regrettably the type which has been occuring in Gloucestershire recently is type B, and against this the vaccine is useless. However there are frequent epidemics of A and C in the sub-Sahara belt of Africa from West Africa across to the Sudan, and in Nepal and Northern India around New Delhi. Recently there have been epidemics in Egypt and Kenya, presumably spreading north and south from the Sudan. It also occurs in the overcrowded conditions of the Haj Pilgrimage in Saudi Arabia, brought in by African Muslims. Only one injection of this vaccine is necessary and it is effective for three years.

Japanese B Encephalitis

Japanese B Encephalitis is an epidemic severe viral disease, spread by mosquitoes which breed in rice fields, and therefore usually occurs only in rural areas. Epidemics occur throughout South East Asia spreading as far west as southern India. The main viral hosts are usually pigs but may also be ducks or birds. It severely affects children and the elderly causing problems in the nervous system. Tourists are rarely affected and only those spending two weeks or more in rural areas in the monsoon season (June to October) require protection. Those living in these areas for a prolonged period should be protected. Two doses are given one to two weeks apart, and in children and the elderly a third injection should be given in four weeks time.

Tick-borne Encephalitis

Tick-borne encephalitis is a similar viral infection of the central nervous system which occurs in forest areas of Central Europe, namely Austria, West Germany, Yugoslavia, Czechoslavia and also the U.S.S.R. and Scandinavia. It mainly affects forestry workers but campers and orienteers could develop it. Two doses four to twelve weeks apart are required for protection. July to October is the worst season.

Tuberculosis

Tuberculosis is common in many parts of the developing world due to overcrowding and poverty. Immunisation must be considered for those going to live in the developing world. All children who have not been immunised with B.C.G. vaccination must be skin tested and if susceptible must be given B.C.G.

Most adults now in the U.K. are not at risk due to immunisation in childhood but they should also be skin tested, and if susceptible be immunised. There must be an interval of at least three weeks between B.C.G. vaccination and the giving of a live vaccine such as yellow fever or polio. No other immunisation should be given in the B.C.G. arm for three months.

Diphtheria

Diphtheria is still common in parts of the developing world. Most travellers do not need protection because immunisation of children in the U.K. has been carried out routinely now for well over 40 years. For non-immunised adults there is a special low-dose vaccine.

It is essential for all necessary immunisations to be carried out well before the journey, with the exception of cholera and gamma globulin due to their short validity. To leave the immunisation programme to the last minute may well invite unnecessary anxiety and even physical upset.

Since going to press an outbreak of Cholera has occurred in Ecuador and Peru.

Vaccinations Required under International Health Regulations

Vaccination	Where required	How long before valid	Length of validity	Min. age	Other comments
Cholera	Generally certain countries in Asia and Africa if arriving within 5 days after leaving infected area. A very few countries in these areas demand it of everyone	6 days	6 months	Usually 1 year. Some countries have no minimum age or less than 1 year	One injection is sufficient
Yellow Fever	Central Africa 15°N to 10°S, Central America from northern border of Panama State to 15°S, but including Bolivia and excluding part of Eastern Brazil	10 days	10 years	Usually 1 year. A few countries have no minimum age limit or less than 1 year	Not at same time as other live vaccines except polio; preferably not in pregnancy. Never to anyone suffering from Hodgkins Disease, leukaemia or AIDS. Polio at same time or three weeks apart

Medically recommended vaccinations

Vaccination	Where advised	Course programme	Validity	Min. age	Other comments
Typhoid	Everywhere except north-west Europe, Canada, northern U.S.A., Australia and New Zealand	Two injections preferably 4 weeks apart — can be 2-8 weeks	Booster every 3 years	2 years	One injection gives short term cover
Tetanus	Everywhere	3 injections 2nd 4-6 weeks after 1st 3rd 6-12 months later	In U.K. Booster every 10 years Travellers Booster every 5 years	NIL	
Poliomyelitis	Everywhere	3 oral doses at monthly intervals	Booster every 5 years for Travellers	NIL	Never to AIDS sufferers. At same time as yellow fever or three weeks apart
Gamma Globulin for hepatitis A	Countries where sanitation is poor — basically as for typhoid	1 injection	2—6 months depending on dose given	NIL	Efficacy proven: does NOT spread AIDS
Plague	Upland and mountainous areas of Africa and South America	2 doses 4 weeks apart; 3rd dose 4-12 weeks later	6 months	1 year	Efficacy poor. Reaction may be severe
Rabies	Backpackers in rural areas Africa, Asia and Americas	2 doses 4 weeks apart; 3rd dose 1 year later	1 year	NIL	If bitten follow up treatment is essential

Medically recommended vaccinations

Vaccination	Where advised	Course programme	Validity	Minimum age	Other comments
Hepatitis B (Engerix B)	All expatriates. Backpackers. Anyone touring for 6 months or more. Health workers anywhere.	2 doses 1 month apart, 3rd dose 6 months later; or 3 doses 1 month apart and 4th dose 12 months later.	5 years	3 years	Essential where medical facilities may be substandard
Meningococcal Meningitis	Sub-Sahara Africa Northern India, Nepal. Saudi Arabia at time of Haj Pilgrimage. Epidemics do occur elsewhere e.g. Egypt, Sudan, Kenya	One injection	3 years	NIL	Under 2 years immune response is less.
Japanese B Encephalitis	Rural areas South East Asia, Indian Sub-continent to Japan incl. Taiwan and Korea (monsoon period)	2 doses 1-2 weeks apart. Children and elderly 3rd dose 4 weeks later	1 year	NIL	Children and elderly have the disease more seriously.
Tick-borne Encephalitis	Forested areas of Central Europe, southern Scandinavia, Western U.S.S.R.; particularly Austria; Seasonal June —October	2 doses 4 weeks apart. 3rd dose 9-12 months later	Up to 6 years	NIL	Avoid Tick bites by wearing thick long socks and heavy shoes

Medically recommended vaccinations

Vaccination	Where advised	Course programme	Validity	Minimum age	Other comments
Diphtheria	Residents in tropical countries with overcrowding and poor hygiene	Special low dose vaccine for non-immunised adults	—	—	For those over 50 living in risk areas
B.C.G. for tuberculosis	Residents in tropical countries with overcrowding and poor hygiene. Non-immune children	One injection. Previous testing for immunity essential	Probably life	NIL	No live vaccine for 3 weeks after B.C.G. No other injections in B.C.G. arm for 3 months

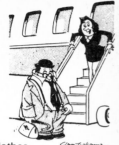

3

Advice for the journey by air or sea

Wear loose-fitting clothes

Both to the experienced and to the less initiated traveller a journey can cause a lot of excitement. Excitement is a mental process and excess can cause mental fatigue. It is bad to start a journey fatigued whether it is by air or sea: whenever possible all preparations should be completed several days before departure, and in particular vaccinations and immunisations should be completed well in advance.

The person who is going abroad for a long time naturally wants to have one or more farewell parties. If possible one should try and have the last of them at least two days before departure because two nights of good sleep before the journey is an excellent principle and, into the bargain, the slightly rarefied atmosphere of the aircraft cabin does not help a "hangover".

Nowadays jet air travel is extremely comfortable but certain factors which can cause temporary discomfort can nearly always be avoided by using a little common sense.

Jet aircraft fly above the bad weather, thus ensuring a far smoother flight than in the old piston-engined aircraft. One of the good points of this is the great decrease in air sickness, or motion sickness as it should be called, but this is discussed more fully shortly.

Effects of pressurisation

Because jet aircraft are at a great height they are flying in a rarefied atmosphere which would not provide sufficient oxygen to maintain life.

Before the days of pressurised cabins aircraft flew below 12,000 feet and hit all the bad weather. Flying above this level in a non-pressurised cabin causes symptoms due to lack of oxygen or "hypoxia". This leads to mental anxiety, lack of co-ordination and judgement, lassitude, sleepiness and disturbance of vision. In the end loss of consciousness or even death will ensue.

As the jet engine flies most economically at over 30,000 feet it is obvious that the cabin must be "pressurised". For this the cabin is completely sealed and the air from the surrounding atmosphere is pumped through the engine compressors. During this process the air is heated to about 500°C, so ridding it of water vapour. This regrettably makes the air in the cabin very dry, causing dehydration in passengers and crew.

Due to technical reasons the atmosphere inside the cabin cannot be maintained as at sea level. For this to be obtained the fuselage would have to be greatly strengthened and the weight would be impractical. As such the usual cabin altitude, as it is called, is between 6,000 and 8,000 feet (but interestingly in Concorde, which is flying even higher, it is maintained at 5,000 - 6,000 feet). As such the air is slightly thinner than at sea level. The pressure of gas is universally proportional to the volume in a confined space. Hence, at 6,000 feet 100 mls of air will increase to 130 mls. This has no harmful effect on the passenger but gases in the body, especially in the intestines, will expand accordingly and an increase of 30 per cent can be quite critical so far as intestinal distension and discomfort is concerned as well as causing earache if one has a cold.

Hence it is inadvisable to eat to excess in an aircraft. Because of the problem of intestinal gases expanding it is a good thing to wear comfortable loose-fitting clothes.

Similarly, if someone is flying with a severe cold and their nose is blocked, they cannot equalise the pressures in their sinuses or ears, and may get sinus pain or earache. Nasal drops or a nasal inhaler may be beneficial on these occasions. A nasal inhaler such as VICK is probably easier to use and less obvious.

Dehydration

As already mentioned the atmosphere in the modern airliner cabin is comparatively dry. Because of this dry atmosphere and the fact that passengers in flight tend not to maintain their fluids a certain degree of dehydration occurs. This is particularly bad for travellers bound for hot climates because dehydration is detrimental to satisfactory acclimatisation to the heat, and therefore must be avoided. With dehydration an uncomfortable dryness of the eyes, nose and/or throat may be noticeable. To prevent this, fluids should be maintained as much as possible on the aircraft. However, because of the tendency for intestinal gases to expand, it is advisable to avoid fizzy or carbonated drinks. Unfortunately alcohol is known to have a bad effect on acclimatisation as it causes dehydration in itself, and so must be kept down to a minimum. As well as alcohol, strong tea and coffee encourage dehydration. All three of these substances act on the kidneys so that more fluid is passed in your urine than you have actually drunk, thus making you more dehydrated.

Smoking

Another problem associated with the slight decrease of oxygen occurs when smoking. Airlines are now providing separate non-smoking and smoking areas which is an excellent idea. Smokers have a certain amount of carbon monoxide in their blood. At a cabin altitude of 6,000 feet, and because of the slight lack of oxygen, this amount of carbon monoxide increases so that a heavy smoker may get early symptoms of excess carbon monoxide; not serious, but enough to cause a headache and discomfort. As such, smoking in flight should be discouraged.

Inactivity

Sitting in the same position for many hours on a long-distance flight causes some venous congestion particularly in the legs, especially if the traveller already suffers from varicose veins. With this problem some minimal swelling of the feet and even the ankles may occur. It may be just enough to cause tightness of the shoes. To prevent this it is a good thing to take a walk up and down the cabin. Recent research work has shown that small doses of aspirin are considered beneficial in preventing blood clots. It would be sensible for passengers with varicose veins to take half an aspirin night and morning in flight provided that they have no history of gastric or duodenal ulcer. Regrettably, with today's security precautions, in general one is not allowed to get out at transit stops, which would give the passengers a little beneficial exercise. The answer then is to wear loose-fitting shoes as well as loose-fitting clothes and to avoid the modern elastic-sided boot or shoe. Lace-up shoes can be loosened and should therefore be your choice. If an overnight flight is being undertaken then it is a good thing to have a comfortable pair of slippers in your night bag. It is sensible for men to take off their ties and undo their collar.

The right clothing

Another problem with clothing is the rapid change of climate which can occur in modern jet travel. One can leave the winter of England one evening and reach the tropics of Africa the next morning and vice versa. Besides this, one must remember that in many parts of the tropics and subtropics there can be far greater variation in temperature over 24 hours than there is in a temperate climate, particularly so in the countries around the the Arabian Gulf. It is therefore essential to have something light and warm at hand for the evening.

Motion sickness

Motion sickness is now a rare occurrence amongst air travellers. Air sickness, sea sickness, car sickness and even travel sickness are all misnomers because it can occur without travelling. Swings, and to a lesser extent, roundabouts are also a major cause.

The history of motion sickness in man dates back as far as the writers of Greek mythology. In fact the word nausea comes from the Greek word *naus* meaning a ship, from which is also derived the word nautical. Throughout history there have been many famous men who have suffered from motion sickness. Probably the first recorded sufferer was Julius Caesar and since then there have been Admiral Nelson and Charles Darwin. To stress the point of motion sickness one can add that Lawrence of Arabia is reported as having suffered from it whilst riding a camel.

Briefly, what causes it? A great many doctors, physiologists and other research workers have tried to find the definitive answer but as yet with only partial success.

It is known that the basic factor is the upset of the labyrinth mechanism in the inner ear, which is part of the organ of balance. This upset is caused by change in acceleration, whether it be linear or angular. The onset of sea sickness with the roll or pitch of the boat is typical of change in angular acceleration. The important aspect of this labyrinthine upset is head movement. If the head remains still, then the effect of these changes in acceleration on the labyrinth is minimised.

As well as the physical cause, there are strong psychological factors such as anxiety and excitement. Many a child who is car sick going away on holiday is well on the journey home.

What is the frequency? Far less than the general public thinks. Lederer and Kidera, two doctors with two American airlines, reckoned in 1954, in the days of piston aircraft flying through bad weather that in one million passengers only 0.5 per cent were sick, — one in two hundred. Today's jet aircraft fly far above the bad weather ensuring a smoother flight, and so the incidence now is around one in a thousand passengers or 0.1 per cent.

How does one prevent it? Those who suffer should avoid sitting in the tail of the aircraft or over the wheels in a bus. In sea travel they should try to remain amidships, and lie down whenever possible. Try to keep the head as still as possible, leaning it against the seat headrest in an aircraft. Do not look out of the window at moving objects. A simple diet with avoidance of fried or fatty foods is sensible, as also is avoidance of excessive alcohol before departure. Avoid smoking, as the smell of smoke may aggravate it. Habitual use of one form of transport is known to cut down the incidence.

There are various tablets which are frequently beneficial in preventing motion sickness. Hyoscine is the principle basis of many of these, of which Kwells is one of the best known. Kwells is frequently effective with children if taken in the recommended dosage. However, although it can be bought over the chemist's counter, it is dangerous if taken to excess. As it is a tasteless tablet great care must be taken to keep it out of the reach of children.

Of the other recommended drugs, most are anti-histamines or are allied to this group. In general they have a mild sedative action as well, which helps with the anxiety factor. Of these the following are effective (the proprietary names in brackets): Cyclizine (Marzine); diphenhydramine (Dramamine); meclozine (Bonamine, Postafine, Sealegs); promethazine (Avomine, Phenergan).

This list is not in order of efficacy and what suits one person may not suit another. It is up to your doctor to choose what he or she thinks, in the circumstances, is best. Care must always be taken with the taking of tablets in pregnancy but again your doctor will advise. Recently yachtsmen have found Stugeron to be effective.

Motion sickness is easier to prevent than to cure, so the first dose must be given at least one hour before the journey and the subsequent doses should be taken according to the advice of your doctor.

Time zone changes

Finally with regard to air travel one must look at the problem that is called jet lag but what in the medical world is called the upset of your circadian (around 24 hours) or diurnal (daytime) rhythms.

With this problem the rapid crossing of time zones when flying east-west or west-east upsets certain of your physiological rhythms.

For every 15 meridians of longitude that are crossed the time changes by one hour. When it is 12 noon G.M.T. in London, it is 4 a.m. in San Francisco, 7 a.m. in New York, 7.30 p.m. in Singapore and 10 p.m. in Sydney. A mid-morning flight from London in a Jumbo arrives shortly after lunch in New York, when according to your body's reckoning it should be late afternoon. This makes a particularly long day.

An overnight flight to the East cuts down the period of darkness so making a short night. These points lead to fatigue problems plus other physiological upsets which are short lasting but must be considered.

These problems are linked to the daily rhythms of the body called circadian, from the Latin *circa* meaning around, and *dies* the day, or in other words around the clock. Sleeping, waking, eating and the emptying of your bowels and bladder are all essentials in daily life which become time controlled.

A great deal of research has been done on this problem during the last 30 years in both the U.S.A. and the U.K. In Oklahoma City, Hauty and Adams, two American doctors, carried out various physiological and psychological tests on a group of fit young men before and after they made three separate flights. First they flew from Oklahoma to Manila, which is flying west, and back after a stay of eight days there. Secondly they flew from Oklahoma to Rome, which is flying east, with a similar stay in Rome before return. Thirdly they flew from Washington D.C. south to Santiago, Chile, and a similar return. In the physiological tests body temperature, pulse rate, breathing rate, and water loss by evaporation were measured. Psychological tests included reaction time, decision time, tests for subjective fatigue and one called the critical flicker fusion time.

It was found that when someone flew north-south or vice versa, none of these factors was upset, except for subjective fatigue, which is only natural after a long flight.

After the flight from Oklahoma to Manila, or in other words flying west, when there was a time displacement of ten hours, the body temperature and the pulse rate were upset for four days. Body temperature is normally highest in the evening about 6 p.m. The test disclosed that during the first 24 hours after flight it was highest at 12 noon, and it did not return to an evening peak for four days. The upset in pulse rate was for the same length of time. The evaporative water loss, which again is time controlled, was upset for eight days. More important, efficiency tests such as reaction, decision, and flicker fusion times were slowed for two days, which meant wrong decisions were being made.

On the Oklahoma—Rome flight, or flying east, the body temperature timing was upset for six days, the pulse rate for eight days, and the evaporative water loss for 12 days. The reaction, decision, and flicker fusion times were slowed for three days. In other words, with flying east the effect was 50 per cent more than with flying west, although in fact the time displacement was seven hours instead of ten hours. With both east and west flights, return to normality after the home-bound flight to Oklahoma was within one day.

Colonel J.M. Adam of the British Army Research team flew a group of paratroopers to Singapore where there is a 7½-hour time change on London G.M.T. For the first three days they passed urine according to English time. Normally urine is passed from approximately 6.30 a.m. to around 11 p.m. depending on the exact hours of getting up and going to bed; add seven and a half hours to match Singapore time, and you get 2 p.m. to 6.30 a.m. He found that, decreasing over the first three days, they were passing two thirds of their urine during the night hours and one third during the day. This naturally caused disturbed sleep, added to their journey fatigue, and lowered their efficiency.

Colonel Adam's colleagues tested 60 paratroopers, again before and after a flight to Singapore, where they were marching, digging, staging assaults, handling weapons and shooting. All tests showed a deterioration in efficiency during the first three days, except in tests where pure military training could have overcome the problem of time change.

Along with the passing of urine, regular bowel habits may be upset for a few days. The person who normally opens his bowels at approximately the same time every day, whether it be on rising, after breakfast or in the evening, may become constipated initially until his bowel clock has become used to the new time. It is therefore advisable to take a mild aperient in your travel case for use, if necessary, after long flights. As your intestinal tract rests during your night hours it is sensible to avoid meals, certainly on the aircraft, and for the first 24 hours after arrival during these hours.

Even more important the sleep pattern may be disturbed for the first few nights. If you fly to New York and go to bed at midnight New York time, you are retiring at 5 a.m. London G.M.T. when your "physiological clock" would normally be preparing to wake you. The answer is to go to bed as near your true home bedtime as possible. In other words, if you went to bed at 9 p.m. in New York it would be 2 a.m. if you were still in London. This may not be perfect but it is better than midnight and 5 a.m.

Try to plan your journey so that you arrive at your final destination — your hotel or house — as near as possible to your normal bedtime (at your point of departure, not your point of arrival). To return to the 9 p.m. — 2 a.m. New York example, of course it would preferably be 7 p.m. and midnight but that might be considered antisocial. To avoid initial sleep problems, it is advisable, having consulted your doctor, to take a mild quick-acting sedative with you. One or two nights use can rid you of any trouble, and by no means encourages a sleeping-pill habit. Remember alcohol should not be taken at the same time as a sleeping pill.

Naturally the older traveller takes longer to re-establish his physiological rhythms than the younger.

The most important thing is that it is wrong to make a trans-Atlantic or equivalent flight and go straight in to an important meeting where major decisions are to be made. For many years politicians of every political colour have met their opposite numbers immediately on arrival with probable dire results. But in 1972 when President Nixon flew to China and Russia he broke his journey en route to rest. In March 1973 when Premier Heath flew to the U.S.A. to see President Nixon he flew over on Saturday to rest on Sunday and see the President on Monday. If common sense is coming even to the politicians, surely we must be able to persuade businessmen.

The business tycoon must never go from the aircraft to the boardroom, as wrong decisions will inevitably be made and this goes for the politician as well. In fact a 24-hour rest period should be ensured whenever there has been a long flight with a five-hour or more time change.

Passengers with special needs

At this stage it is opportune to mention some of the medical conditions which may lead to problems when flying in civil aircraft, but it must be stressed that there are few people who are unfit to fly in modern pressurised wide-bodied jet aircraft. The main factor in causing problems is the minor degree of rarefaction of the air in the pressurised cabin and with it the decrease in oxygen content.

What must be remembered is that the major airlines have medical departments and, if any medical problems are notified to the airline when the reservations are made, then the medical department in association with the passenger's own doctor can give suitable advice, and if necessary, make special arrangements or even provide special diets. It is the "un-notified" handicapped or invalid passenger who can cause a problem both for himself and perhaps for the airline. B.O.A.C., B.E.A. and subsequently British Airways have been leaders in these matters in the airline world.

UNFIT TO FLY

- Patients with infectious diseases in period of infection
- Expectant mothers — after 35th week intercontinental flights
  — after 36th domestic and short haul flight
- Severe anaemia
- Recent heart attack or stroke, or uncontrolled heart failure
- Severe ear or sinus infection, or recent major ear surgery
- Bleeding from stomach ulcer within last 3 weeks
- Within 10 days of simple abdominal surgery
- Within 14 days of chest surgery
- Wired fractures of the jaw
- Mental illness without attendance and sedation

Besides the problems aggravated by altitude and decreased oxygen there can be some physical problems of fitting people into seats. Passengers with lower leg plasters, or fixed hips or knees, may simply not fit in. Even if they can be accommodated they might have to remain in a position of severe discomfort for several hours. It can be said that the front row of seats in the economy class and those in the "emergency exit" rows have more leg room but the front row is usually reserved for mothers with babies in carry-cots, and safety regulations forbid the allocation of emergency row seats to handicapped passengers. In addition one cannot have a plastered leg sticking out into the gangway. The only answer may be to travel first class or on a stretcher.

Obviously the decreased amount of oxygen can affect passengers with heart failure, a recent coronary thrombosis, marked anaemia, or severe respiratory disease with breathlessness. It is also detrimental in elderly people whose hardened arteries and ageing hearts provide only just enough oxygen for the brain under normal circumstances. As a result of the decrease in oxygen they may become confused during long international flights.

So far as the rarefaction of the air is concerned this can affect people with sinus trouble causing sinus pain and earache and those who have stomach or intestinal lesions by causing the expansion of gases. This is particularly so after recent gastric or intestinal operations or haemorrhage.

Diabetes mellitus

There can be problems for diabetics on insulin who are flying long distances with time changes of several hours. For short trips diabetics can ususally select a satisfactory diet from the normal menus but it is essential that they do have at hand reserve carbohydrate in the form of sweets and starch so that they can give themselves first aid if they are becoming hypoglycaemic (fall in blood sugar). On long flights they should ignore the time changes and continue on meal and injection times accordingly to their home time until they arrive at their destination. After arrival each insulin injection can be altered by two or three hours until the current schedule with new local time is reached. With westward travel the time between injections is slightly longer so a small additional dose of soluble insulin may be necessary. With eastward travel the time between injections is slightly less and so the dose of insulin may have to be cut by a few units (4 to 8). The most important point is to test the urine every four to six hours to keep a constant check. With care and common sense normal control should be established within two to three days.

The other important point is that all diabetics on insulin must carry in their hand luggage an ample supply of insulin, needles and syringes, testing equipment and any other personal drugs. Aircraft can be delayed and if these necessities for life are in the hold nothing can be done about it, and anyway insulin must not freeze.

The shelf life of insulin is decreased in hot climates. The British Diabetic Association produces a pamphlet giving advice for the diabetic traveller. Finally the diabetic traveller should inform the airline in advance so suitable meals can be provided at different times if necessary.

Pregnant women and infants

Of the "physiological" problems one must mention pregnancy, children and infants. Regarding pregnancy, motion sickness remedies must not be taken without previous discussion with the passenger's own doctor. Yellow fever vaccination should not be given during pregnancy. The feet and ankles are more likely to swell up at this time. In general, pregnant mothers are accepted for travel on inter-continental flights up to the end of the 35th week of pregnancy (i.e. four weeks before the expected date of birth) provided everything is normal. For shorter flights they are accepted up to the end of the 36th week. Infants in general travel well. The passages in their upper respiratory system are comparatively wider than in adult life and so they have less problems with their ears. If they get earache they cry and this automatically clears the passages. Infants who are still on a four-hourly or equivalent feeding pattern are far less upset by the change in circadian rhythms. Small children also travel well but, for the sake of their parents and other passengers, an adequate supply of forms of amusement for the journey is sound practice.

Contraception

Women passengers on oral contraceptives must remember that in many overseas countries it is against religious principles to sell the pill, and that if the taker is vomiting or has diarrhoea the pill may not be absorbed. Women suffering from hepatitis must not take the pill then or for some time afterwards, depending on the severity of the hepatitis. Medical advice must be sought.

All medicines including anti-malarials, which are going to be taken whilst overseas on a long-term basis are strictly not allowed to be obtained on the N.H.S. They must be purchased on a private prescription.

To summarise, one can say that there are very few people who are unfit to fly in modern jet aircraft and if someone is wanting to travel to a centre for specialist treatment then all airlines will be guided by humanitarian principles.

SUMMARY

Preflight and inflight advice

1 Plan your flight well in advance; if possible take a day flight and/or arrive at your usual bedtime.

2 Not too hectic 24 hours before flight.

3 Try to cut smoking before and in flight.

4 Moderate your alcohol in flight.

5 Moderate your food in flight.

6 Maintain your fluids in flight — avoid sparkling drinks.

7 Wear loose fitting, comfortable clothes and shoes.

8 Keep light but warm clothing at hand.

9 Maintain a 24-hour minimum rest period on arrival after 5-hour time change. Never go straight into a meeting or a reception.

10 Carry a mild aperient and mild quick acting sedative with you if you are crossing time zones.

Travelling by sea

Having discussed the problems of modern air travel let us turn to sea travel. More and more routine travel is by air because of the time factor and the constant rush of present-day life. This is so to such an extent that a large percentage of modern passenger liners spend the majority of their working life cruising. Two or more weeks on a comfortable ship in a warm climate is a wonderful way to get away from it all. Because of this it is now a very popular holiday and a larger percentage of the "cruisers" tend to be in the older age groups, which can cause problems. The major shipping companies have excellent medical departments which have shore-based doctors and nursing staff as well as competent and experienced ships' doctors and nurses. As with the airlines the shipping company's medical department should be informed in advance if elderly, infirm or incapacitated people are travelling by sea. Special arrangements can then be made to help them.

With regard to sunburn at sea, the movement of the ship and a cooling sea breeze with an overcast sky can be very misleading and hence lead to severe burning. However the whole subject of sunburn and its prevention will be discussed in Chapter Five.

As with air travel, swelling of the ankles may occur. This is probably brought on by excessive sitting around in deck chairs, especially in the tropics and sub tropics. Swollen ankles were originally called deck ankles or Colombo flop but sensible exercise helps to clear the condition. A doctor can prescribe pills which will help if it persists.

It is important that any passenger who is at sea for more than a day or two and is on regular medication should have a doctor's letter with them explaining the problem, and also that such patients should take a sufficient supply of their tablets or treatment to last until they get home.

Some of the smaller shipping companies, especially those sailing under flags of convenience, provide only minimal medical facilities. For the elderly or invalid passenger, travel with these companies can cause problems. On some of these cruises passengers who wish to stay on board when shore tours have been arranged are not encouraged. This can be fatiguing for the elderly especially if the weather is hot.

For some passengers there can be problems involved in moving between decks, especially in smaller liners where stairs may be steep and lifts are in unsuitable places. This bars the recent sufferer from a coronary thrombosis.

In general the larger and faster ships are more stable in the water as they are fitted with stabilisers, anti-pitch bow thrusters and up-to-date navigational and safety equipment.

4

Climate and acclimatisation

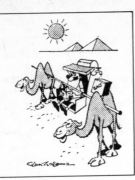

Before air travel, the voyager took many days to go by sea from temperate to warm climates, and then on to tropical climates. With air travel in the jet age, it is quite different. You can be in winter weather in the U.K. one day with temperatures below freezing — anyway at night — and within 24 hours be in the hot and humid climate of Singapore or West Africa. This must create a strain on the human system, if only briefly, until it has become used to it or, as we say, acclimatised. Even in the tropics climates vary. In such as Singapore, Sri Lanka, and the West and East African coasts, it is hot and humid. In the Arabian Gulf and other desert areas it may be even hotter, but it is far less humid and, because of this, the climate is far less trying. In Appendix D at the end of the book there is a brief summary of the climates in various parts of the world.

On sudden transference from the mild or cold weather of Britain to the tropics, the natural body response would be a rise in temperature. However, this rise would be detrimental to the highly sensitive functioning organs of the body. A rise in temperature of 2 to 3°C (3 to 5°F) can be harmful to the highly sensitive brain. There is an area in the brain, called the hypothalamus, where there is a heat regulatory centre which controls two basic mechanisms to keep the body temperature constant, as and when external temperatures rise. The most important is the sweating mechanism, as increased sweating leads to cooling. Many of us at school were lucky — or unlucky — enough to do a little simple physics, and will remember in "heat" how there is a factor called the latent heat of vaporisation. When the sweat vaporises the body loses heat.

The other mechanism is the heart and circulatory system, in which certain basic changes also take place.

What are these basic changes which occur during acclimatisation?

1 Changes in the sweating mechanism:
   (a) Sweating starts at a lower temperature.
   (b) The amount of sweating is greater at any given temperature.
   (c) The body develops an ability to maintain a high production of sweating for longer periods without the sweat glands becoming fatigued.

These three changes together naturally increase the amount of sweating and hence increase the amount of heat lost by the body by the evaporation of this sweat.

2 Changes occur in the blood circulatory system to the surface and the limbs:
   (a) Heat transfer from the body to the surface increases and hence heat is lost by convection.
   (b) Dilation (widening) of the surface blood vessels occurs at a lower temperature than normal.
   (c) The flow of the blood to the skin is higher at any body temperature above normal levels.

3 There is a fall in resting body temperature, thus encouraging the factors mentioned in (1) and (2).

By combining all of the above changes, the body remains cool and is unaffected by the increased heat of the new climate.

It can also be seen that by far the most important factor in the maintainance of a satisfactory temperature in a hot climate is that the body sweats sufficiently. Sweat is basically a salt water solution, and so another vital factor in maintaining satisfactory acclimatisation is the intake of sufficient fluid and salt. The most common cause of failure therefore is failure to maintain these two essentials.

How long does it take to become acclimatised to the new climate? Obviously the extent of difference between the old and the new climate is the biggest factor but, apart from this, much of it occurs within the first week, approximately 80 to 90 per cent within two weeks whilst full acclimatisation probably takes up to six weeks. During the first three days the main strain is on the heart and circulation until the time changes have occurred. On returning to the temperate climate most of the physiological adaptation has been lost within one month. But there is good reason to believe that some effect, possibly a psychological one, is retained by those who have learned by previous experience that, even several years later, they show better adjustment to heat exposure.

What must be remembered by travellers is that, despite what they may think and feel, they sweat just as much in a hot, dry climate as in a hot humid climate. In the latter, as the atmosphere is very nearly saturated with moisture, it is unable to absorb any more of your perspiration, so you remain "bathed in your sweat" as the saying goes. In a dry climate, where the atmosphere is nowhere near saturated, your perspiration evaporates quickly into the atmosphere so that your skin is comparatively dry and you may mistakenly think you have not been sweating.

Altitude acclimatisation

There are several important cities in the world, particularly Nairobi and Johannesburg, which are at an altitude of around 6,000 feet (1,850 metres) whilst Bogotá is at 8,500 feet (2,615 metres). When flying in a pressurised plane at a cabin altitude of 6,000 feet (1,850 metres) you have minor problems, but you are just sitting in your seat nearly all of the time. When, however, you arrive in Nairobi or Johannesburg, you are moving about, and during the first few days you will definitely find you have less "wind". Going up one or two flights of stairs which at home you do easily may well cause breathlessness. The problem is that you are not getting enough oxygen into your lungs because the atmosphere is slightly rarefied. However, your body soon compensates. Because oxygen in the air is taken up by your blood cells you start to make new blood cells, so that there are more in you to grab what oxygen there is.

In general it takes up to three weeks to become acclimatised to the altitude of Nairobi and Johannesburg, but slightly longer for Bogotá. I was asked to advice the British team for the Olympic Games in Mexico which is 7,400 feet (2,275 metres) above sea level. We insisted that they should do no training for the first four days after arrival in Mexico, to allow their circadian rhythms to settle, and it was arranged that they were in Mexico for four weeks before the games, so that they were thoroughly adjusted to the altitude.

However, there are many, mainly younger groups, who wish to go to greater heights. Trekking in Nepal is popular and there are fascinating places to visit at high altitude in the northern part of South America. If you visit Tibet and fly to Lhasa you land at 11,700 feet (3,600 metres) and if you travel by road to the Everest Base Camp you reach 16,900 feet (5,200 metres).

Acute Mountain Sickness is a name given to a collection of complaints or symptoms which commonly occur when people travel to 11,500 feet (3,500 metres). The severity of symptoms and the speed of onset vary greatly in different people and, as might be expected, they are more severe and more frequent in the older and less physically fit. The problems are caused by lack of oxygen and the symptoms are nausea, dizziness, difficulty in sleeping, loss of appetite, headache and fatigue. The traveller has undue breathlessness on exertion, a forcible heart beat and slow sighing breathing when sleeping. The symptoms do not appear for 36 to 48 hours and usually wear off if no further ascent is made. However, with further climbing they may return. Around 50 per cent of travellers will have some of these symptoms at 11,500 feet (3,500 metres) and 80-90 per cent at 16,500 feet (5,000 metres).

Recently a pill (acetazolamide), sold as DIAMOX, has been found to be useful in preventing Acute Mountain Sickness if taken for several days before ascending. One pill of 250 mgm Diamox taken for three days before ascent and continued until 5,000 metres is reached is recommended. Common side effects from Diamox are tingling, pins and needles or numbness in hands and feet.

Remember, far more important than pills is to climb more slowly and, if symptoms occur, to go no higher; or if they get worse, to descend.

Factors affecting acclimatisation

Whether it is acclimatising oneself to heat or to altitude, there are various factors which help or hinder.

1 **Age** — Naturally the younger the adult, the more quickly he or she acclimatises.
2 **Fatigue** — Fatigue definitely slows down the rate of acclimatisation; and thus it is important for the traveller to avoid over-fatigue.
3 **Dehydration** — With increased sweating, it is essential for the individual to take in more fluid than normal, or dehydration will occur, which is the worst state possible for satisfactory acclimatisation.
4 **Obesity** — It has been found that excess weight slows down ability to acclimatise. A general high standard of physical fitness aids rapid acclimatisation.
5 **Sex** — It has been shown that men acclimatise better than women when living under similar conditions. Testosterone, the male hormone, stimulates sweating and it is considered this may be the main reason.

6 **Fever** — Not unnaturally if a newcomer to a tropical area develops an infective fever on arrival the process of acclimatisation is upset.

Helping oneself acclimatise

1 Maintenance of fluids

The maintenance of one's fluid intake in warm climates is so important that it cannot be mentioned too frequently. It must be quite obvious that if maintenance of sweating is the essential in keeping fit in a hot climate, then the constant replacement of salt and water used up in sweating is an absolute 'must'. There are two simple general principles to work on regarding the maintenance of fluids.

● First, in every 24 hours you should drink one pint of fluid for every ten degrees of Fahrenheit temperature. This means that if the temperature is 80°F, then you drink eight pints of fluid between 8 am one morning and 8 am the next morning. If the temperature rises to 100°F, then one has to drink ten pints in the 24 hours. With metrication, one must consider what one would need in litres and degrees centigrade. If one takes a basic two litres in the 24 hours and adds one litre for every 10°C, then the rate of fluid intake is very nearly the same i.e. four litres at 20°C, five litres at 30°C and six litres at 40°C.

● The other simple principle to remember with regard to fluid intake is to see that your urine remains nearly colourless. Once your urine becomes a yellow colour, it means it is concentrating, and you are beginning to be dehydrated. As well as upsetting acclimatisation, dehydration can cause other problems, for prolonged concentration of the urine causes formation of kidney stones, which leads to the painful condition of renal colic.

2. Maintenance of salt

Along with the fluid loss due to increased sweating, there is salt loss which must therefore be replaced as well as fluids. The normal European diet contains about ten grams of salt per 24 hours. In the tropics, because of the sweating, the requirement rises to 15 to 25 grams per 24 hours, depending on the actual heat and the amount of physical work. This therefore means an addition of 5 to 15 grams per day, or on average a doubling of the amount normally taken at home. How can you take this extra salt?

● You can add extra salt to your cooking, and to your food at the table.

● You can put salt in your drinks.

● You can take salt tablets.

● You can combine all three methods.

The main trouble with the taking of salt other than with food is that it tends to make one feel sick, if not actually be sick.

There are two basic types of salt tablet. There is one which is dissolved in water, and it makes an effervescent semi-lemon flavoured drink. It is little different from putting a teaspoonful of salt in a lemon drink. In fact, as it only contains 300 mgm or ⅓ of a gram approximately, there is far less salt in the drink compared with adding salt to lemon squash.

Another type of salt tablet is one known as the enteric coated tablet which means that it passes through the stomach unchanged and dissolves in the enteron or intestine. Because of this property, it does not cause nausea, which is a good point in its favour. This tablet contains 800 mgm of salt which is a far better dose. But each person's bowel acts differently. Studies done in the Royal Air Force showed that patients with rapidly acting intestines have passed these enteric coated tablets undissolved in their motions. This will occur during an attack of diarrhoea when the bowel action is rapid. There is constant loss of fluid and salt in the motions, which is just the time when more salt is needed.

It is thought that by far the best way to take extra salt is to include plenty when cooking and add more to food. It is interesting that under these conditions you are quite happy to eat food which is far more salty than you would eat in temperate climates. You can also add some salt to water or fruit drinks, when again it seems quite palatable.

It was thought that, as acclimatisation takes place, the body's salt loss decreases, resulting in a corresponding decrease in the need for extra salt. However, recent work in the Royal Air Force has shown this to be a fallacy, and the need to continue with extra salt is essential.

What is most important is that whatever you do, you must not raise your salt intake without raising your fluid intake. If you do this, you are in a worse position than if you do not increase them at all. However, if you want to acclimatise yourself successfully and rapidly to a hot climate, you must maintain both your fluids and your salt.

3 Clothing

We all now realise that what is most important in aiding man to acclimatise quickly and well to a new hot, or even warm, climate is the maintenance of satisfactory sweating. We accept that extra fluid and extra salt are necessary to produce sufficient sweat and that the next important step is to encourage evaporation of the sweat to keep the body cool. Obviously no clothes at all would be an answer, but it is not the complete answer. The wearing of clothes is most important for protection against the sun and against insects, thorny plants and snakes. It is also most important to keep as much covered as possible after dusk when mosquitoes bite.

The answer is to wear fabrics which aid absorption of the sweat and loose clothes, so that there is a layer of air between the skin and the clothing which aids evaporation. Remember also that a layer of air between your clothes and skin keeps you warm in the cold and cool in the heat. Tight gloves give you cold fingers and tight shoes cold toes. Having decided your clothing must be loose-fitting the next thing one must decide is what are the best materials.

Choosing materials which encourage acclimatisation

Clothes must be loose and light in weight. Previous work done by one of the Medical Research Council teams reckoned that every kilogram (2.2lb) of clothes worn, was the equivalent of raising the temperature 1°C (or 1.8°F). It is also important for clothes to be light in colour, as this reflects heat, whilst dark clothes absorb the heat.

It has been shown with people working in the sun that white clothing can reduce the solar heat load by 50 per cent.

Hence clothes should be loose, light in weight and light in colour.

The final but most important point is that the material of the clothing must be capable of absorbing the sweat so as to encourage further sweating. The material with the highest absorbent properties is wool but this is too thick and heavy for warm climates. Next on the list in absorptive properties is rayon which absorbs at least 70 per cent of its weight in water, but is similarly unsatisfactory for wear in the tropics. After this comes cotton which is by far the best material for tropical wear. It absorbs 50 per cent of its weight in water, or in other words one pound of cotton clothing will absorb half a pound of water.

But what of all the man-made fibres developed during the last few years with all their drip dry and non-crease properties? To the traveller, especially the businessman going round the world in two or three weeks, the arrival of drip dry shirts and socks was a tremendous boon.

But what makes the material "drip dry" is its inability to absorb water, known as the water inhibition characteristic, so that microscopically the water remains on the surface, therefore these materials are not suitable when sweating is high and needs to be encouraged.

The absorptive properties of the man-made fibres are as follows:

Modacrylic (Dynel and Teklan)	15—20%
Triacetates (Aranel, Rhonel, Tricel)	10—11%
Acrylic (Acrilan, Courtelle, Dralon, Orlon)	8—11%
Metallic (Lurex)	5%
Nylon (Brinylon, Celon, Enkalon, Penlon, Ribson)	4—12%
Elastofibre (Lycra, Sponzelle)	3%
Polyester (Dacron, Terylene, Trevira)	3%

If they are to be worn in the pure state in the tropics the manufacturers should develop minute perforations in the material so that perspiration can pass through.

"Drip dry" cotton shirts are available but after several washings they lose this property, because they have been treated with resins which have made them drip dry by removing the absorptive properties. As this resin is washed out, absorption improves and drip-dry properties decrease. As such, a truly-drip dry cotton shirt is not a great deal better than some man-made fibres.

From this one can see that if one wears pure man-made fibres next to the skin, one will remain literally in a pool of sweat which encourages prickly heat. If one cannot wear pure cotton the answer is to wear a mixture with more cotton than man-made fibre. A small percentage of man-made fibre will definitely increase the wearing properties of the clothes as also the crease resistance. It must be remembered with socks that this percentage must be small. Pure nylon socks will cause the feet to be sweaty and smelly.

Wearing hats

During the 1914—1918 war, the "solar topee" was considered to be absolutely essential for any European in the tropics. Women, whenever they were allowed in the tropics, wore either similar topees, or wide-brimmed hats. At that time it was incorrectly thought that all heat disturbances were prevented by wearing a hat. We now know that most heat disturbances are prevented by maintaining one's fluid and salt.

An interesting point is that it is now known that the head area provides 25 per cent of the total sweat area of the body and so it is important that it is not covered unnecessarily.

In dry desert areas, where sweating is easy and sweat evaporates, the sun streams out of a clear sky and initially it is probably wise to wear a hat. In humid climates where evaporation of sweat is more difficult and the sky is usually overcast, thus preventing glare, it is probably best not to wear a hat.

Underwear

Some prefer to wear and others prefer to be without underwear. The basic principle is that a layer of air between the shirt or blouse and the skin is good both for warmth and for coolness.

On this principle, it is best to wear cotton string vests and pants when travelling from one climate to another. String vests keep you cool in the tropics and warm in the cold of a European winter.

SUMMARY

Acclimatisation

1 Avoid fatigue.
2 Maintain your fluids: 1 pint per 10°F per 24 hours.
3 Maintain your salt: preferably add salt to your food.
4 Never wear nylon in the heat.
5 Climb slowly: if symptoms of mountain sickness occur climb no further.

Keeping fresh

Clean underwear, shirts and socks daily are obviously essential in the tropics. It is fine if you can change them once in the morning and a second time after showering or bathing, after work for the evening. If you can put clean clothing on only once a day it is best to do so after work for the evening when you sweat less, so your clothes are still fresh for the morning.

Therefore the main points in aiding you to acclimatise are to avoid fatigue, maintain your fluids and salt, and dress sensibly.

5

Heat disorders

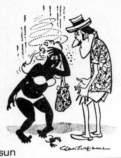

Go easy on the sun

There are certain problems which may beset the newcomer to the tropics but if he or she has carried out the suggestions made in the previous chapter, there is no need to suffer from any of them at any time.

In addition to the advice already given, remember that if you develop a temperature because of influenza, malaria, dysentery or any other illness, it is an added strain on the body's temperature control system. More care must be taken to correct a fever in the tropics than in a temperate climate. In other words, your fluid and salt intake must be increased even more than they have been already.

Heat disorders

Probably the classic incidence of heat disorder was the Black Hole of Calcutta in 1756, when 123 out of 146 died after being imprisoned for one night.

Satisfactory acclimatisation naturally minimises the risk of subsequent heat disorders.

Heat syncope; heat collapse; or exercise-induced heat exhaustion

These are different names for the same condition which probably in its mildest form is about the most common and unpleasant response to sudden heat, its suddenness being the most important point. In general, it occurs in those recently arrived and unacclimatised but with the acclimatised long-term resident or "local", it only occurs with a sudden change in temperature and in particular, a rise in humidity. It is reported that a group of Arab road-builders in Kuwait suffered from it in a sudden heatwave, so it is not confined to the visitor.

In its mildest form, symptoms are light-headedness or dizziness in hot surroundings and mainly with a change of position. Fainting may occur, especially if excess exercise is undertaken and there may also be generalised and acute fatigue, nausea, yawning and blurring of vision.

Treatment consists of brief rest, fluid and salt. It usually means the sufferer has done too much before becoming acclimatised.

Heat hyperpyrexia and heat stroke

These are the most serious and acute disorders affecting anyone in the tropics. Heat hyperpyrexia means that the body temperature rises to 105°F or even higher, due to a failure of the heat regulation control. The same occurs in heat stroke, but as well as the marked rise in temperature, the sufferer becomes unconscious. Both are due to the sudden failure of the sweating mechanism from water depletion because the person has not drunk enough to provide for the excess sweating; whilst a concurrent raised temperature puts too much load on the sweating mechanism so that the sweat glands cease to work. Excess clothes or exercise can provoke the condition. The initial symptoms suggest heat collapse but they worsen, the temperature rises, the skin becomes dry and hot, and unconsciousness may ensue.

If people behave sensibly this condition is rare, but if it does occur, expert medical attention is necessary. However, time is a definite factor, and simple first aid treatment can be started before a doctor arrives. The spraying of the skin of the patient's entire body with water cooled to 12—15°C (54—59°F) in a stream of dry air is best, in contrast with immersion in a cold bath; when the cooling is less controlled.

Wrapping in a wet sheet is effective but the patient's temperature must be taken at least every five minutes and, when the rectal temperature has fallen to 102°F, all cooling methods must be stopped, else collapse may ensue due to excess cooling.

It is unlikely that the ordinary business traveller or holidaymaker will experience this condition but the expatriate, working manually in intense heat, must be vigilant.

Heat oedema

This is swelling of the ankles due to heat, which may occur in the first week or ten days, and is also known as deck ankles, from the days when travellers had their first experience of the tropics whilst still at sea, or Colombo flop. It is more common in women, and disappears in a few days, but its disappearance is helped by cutting down on standing and walking.

The two other main heat disorders are those due to either salt or water depletion.

Salt depletion

This shows itself mainly with fatigue, giddiness, muscle cramps, and vomiting and it takes about three to five days to develop.

If heavy exercise is taken when there is a minor degree of salt depletion, intense muscle cramps are frequent.

Treatment is to take drinks as heavily-salted as possible without causing vomiting. As vomiting is sometimes a symptom of salt depletion, it can be a problem, and if it continues, medical advice must be sought because it may be necessary for salted fluids to be given by means other than by mouth. Consommé, beef tea, tomato juice, and fruit juices are suitable vehicles with which to cover up the taste of salt and the sufferer should rest in the cool.

Water depletion

Symptoms, which can develop within only one to three days of fluid lack, are intense thirst, diminishing sweating, urine which is highly concentrated and small in volume, and sometimes a raised temperature. Pain in the loins and on passing urine may ensue. Treatment consists of as much fluid as possible such as 12 pints in the first 24 hours. As the body temperature rises with water depletion cool sponging may be necessary.

It is obvious that all the above general effects of excess heat can be avoided by common sense. Namely:

1   Avoid excess physical fatigue during the period of acclimatisation.

2   Maintain fluids: at least one pint to every 10°F per 24 hours; or with Celsius readings, a basis of 2 litres, and in addition one litre for every 10°C = 4 litres at 20°C and 5 litres at 30°C etc.

3   Maintain salt intake by adding extra salt to the food. This is particularly important during the period of acclimatisation.

4   What is most important is that you must not increase your salt without increasing your fluids.

Joseph   Banks,   the   distinguished   naturalist   of   the eighteenth century who was subsequently President of the Royal Society, accompanied Captain James Cook on his first visit to Tahiti. In his writings in the *Journal of the Endeavour* (1768—1771) he described a dinner given by the Tahitians. Everyone was given one half coconut shell of ordinary water and one of salted water. The Tahitians obviously had the answer: on taking extra salt, they doubled their fluid intake.

Skin disorders

In addition to these generalised disorders due to heat, there are also skin disorders due to heat which are equally preventable.

Prickly heat

This irritating skin rash usually occurs in the early days after arrival in the tropics or semi-tropics. In 1953 the number of cases in the British Army personnel in Singapore rose sharply to a peak following four to five months' exposure. The rash is caused by the the blocking of the sweat glands leading to the formation of small red blisters on a mildly pink skin. The areas most likely to be affected are the front of the elbows and forearms, over the breast bone and collarbone, around the waist — especially in the belt area, in the armpits and behind the knees. In other words, in hollows and where clothes press against the skin. So sweat remains without evaporating and pooling occurs.

Sogginess of the skin is the prime factor in the beginning of this condition. What causes this sogginess?

Humidity results in the inability of sweat to evaporate because the atmosphere is already saturated whilst clothes prevent the sweat either evaporating or being absorbed. What clothes help sweat to evaporate? Loose-fitting clothes and string vests create the essential layer of air between the clothes and the skin which encourages evaporation and the prevention of prickly heat. What clothes prevent absorption? Pure nylon and other man-made fibres which have no absorptive properties at all. Cotton is the material of choice but it may have a small percentage of man-made fibre in it to improve the wearing properties.

The other important factor in preventing prickly heat is the provision of suitable air-conditioning in hot and humid climates. It has been found that if there is adequate air-conditioning in bedrooms giving eight hours sleep in 24 hours, and thus allowing sweat to evaporate, the sweat glands will rarely block.

If prickly heat does occur how does one treat it?
- Get rid of all man-made fibre clothing.
- Bath without soap and dry well.

● Apply calamine lotion or a dusting powder to clean dry skin. To avoid infection of the blisters, the use of Phisomed (hexachlorophane 3% in detergent base) lotion is effective. An astringent lotion of 95% alcohol with 1 in 2,000 mercuric chloride tones the skin. Most male after-shave and body lotions are fairly similar, and can be used with effect. Loose-fitting clothes must be used subsequently to prevent recurrence.

Prickly heat normally responds rapidly to these simple medicaments. Problems usually only occur on the rare occasions when the mouth becomes infected, and then medical advice should be sought, as an antibiotic may well be necessary.

Sunburn

Sunburn — technically known as acute solar or actinic dermatitis and solar erythema — is the second skin problem which may occur in the heat.

Initially sunburn shows itself as a simple reddening of the skin, but in severe cases the skin becomes swollen, thickened, and tender, while later blistering may occur.

By now there are usually constitutional signs such as headache, general malaise, nausea and sometimes vomiting; and the skin is extremely tender and the sufferer unable to bear the weight of clothes on the skin, or is unable to lie down and rest. With severe burning, high fever can ensue and fatalities have been known, although general reactions usually last only a few hours.

Here again, this is an entirely preventable condition. In the services, sunburn is considered an offence due to self-neglect. Initially there should only be short exposure in the form of sunbathing. I very much regret that the average Englishman is very foolish on sudden arrival on the Mediterranean and other shores, for his annual holiday in the sun. The majority of visitors to warmer climates are only away for a maximum of two weeks, and some for an even shorter period, with the result that they frequently strip off and lie out in the sun, straightaway after arrival, for long periods.

For anyone going to semi-tropical and tropical shores from the U.K. 15 minutes is plenty of time for the first "sunning" session. After this, it can be increased daily to 30 minutes, one hour, two hours, three hours and then an extra hour per day, until at the end of two weeks they can be lying out all day.

A great deal of work has been done by the medical profession over the last few years concerning the incidence of skin cancer following excessive sun exposure. There is now strong evidence that natural sunlight is the main factor in causing certain cancers (basal cell and squamous cell carcinoma). This evidence relates to long-term exposure to sunlight generally in an occupational setting. With these two types of cancer the outlook is excellent, if diagnosed and treated early, as they are generally only locally malignant.

Surveys from the U.S.A., South Africa and Australia have shown that the incidence of these types of skin cancer are far commoner in white skinned people living in the lower latitudes e.g. Texas, South Africa and Australia.

However with the far more serious type of skin cancer, the malignant melanoma which can spread internally, evidence would suggest that short term exposure to intense sunlight of skin which is not normally exposed is the most important factor in this group of malignancies. What has also been found is that these serious malignancies are far commoner in people with light brown or blonde hair, blue eyes and fair skin and pigmented moles.

People who are taking steroids must also be particularly careful. After a blistering sunburn or redness remaining for more than a week, trouble may occur. It definitely appears that these melanomas have an increased incidence in people who have suffered sunburn episodes in the last five years. All of these problems are rarer in dark skinned people.

Sunbathing which exceeds greater exposure than the lengths of time already mentioned is asking for trouble, even when using good creams and lotions. Care must also be taken in the purchase of these because the less well-known makes may contain filtering factors which can cause unpleasant skin sensitivities.

Recently, new suntanning lotions and creams have been produced containing bergamot oil. One active principle of this oil is a substance called 5-methoxy-psoralen which promotes tanning with ultraviolet light. Some medical authorities maintain that it is not prudent to incorporate psoralen into suntan preparations while others consider that as the psoralen promotes tanning it is beneficial in preventing further damage from the sun's rays.

Over 30 years ago a preparation containing Vitamin A and calcium carbonate in a pill was produced in South Africa which was claimed to be beneficial in preventing the pain of sunburn without upsetting the tanning effect of the sun. It is sold under the name of Sylvasun and first became available in the U.K. in 1968, although it had been used by the British Olympic teams before then and most of the athletes felt it was helpful.

The author with two colleagues carried out an extensive trial of Sylvasun in 1970 involving over 1,600 people who were on holiday mainly in the Mediterranean area and the tropics. Of 640 self-classified as severe or moderate burners, 90 per cent felt they were substantially helped by Sylvasun. Regrettably, for administrative reasons, it was not possible to carry out the trial using a "control" group (50 per cent having a "dud" pill or placebo) so there has been criticism of its efficiency. At no time has any responsible body suggested that Sylvasun taken in the recommended dosage was toxic or had any side effects; but equally one must say that there is no evidence that its use has any beneficial or detrimental effect on the prevention of skin cancer.

It is my opinion that if Sylvasun can be obtained, it is worth taking two pills a day for the first two weeks of exposure, but creams and lotions must still be used and exposure time not altered. However, Sylvasun should not be taken in pregnancy. If Sylvasun is not available (as is now the state of affairs in the U.K.) then Roavit capsules (which are Vitamin A alone), one daily, can be used instead.

Special care is needed with the auburn-haired, who were found to be the most susceptible. The fair-haired and fair-skinned person burns easily, but they are greatly helped by Sylvasun, which does not seem to be so helpful with the auburn-haired

In preventing excessive sunburn the power of reflected light must be remembered. Very light sand, a clear sea, and the snow of winter sports all reflect a great deal of the sun's rays, so making its ultimate effect far greater than is realised.

There is a small percentage of people who are highly sensitive to the sun and who cannot expose their skin without severe skin reactions. For these people the only answer is the use of a barrier cream. This, of course, prevents any trouble, but as it is a barrier, the user naturally does not tan. Such a cream is Uvistat, made by Ward Blenkinsop, of which the active ingredient is mexenone 4%. If used in very small quantities it can be only a partial barrier and then some tanning may occur. The manufacturer also produces Uvistat-L, which is a similar sunburn-protecting lip salve. More recently other preparations like Uvistat have been available through the N.H.S. All reputable sun creams and lotions now have a Sunburn Protection Factor (S.P.F.), indicated by number on the bottle which can be more than 20. Anybody who is liable to sunburn should use a preparation with an S.P.F. above 6. It is possible that these preparations also prevent or delay the development of premature ageing changes and pre-cancerous and cancerous skin damage. All creams and lotions need frequent application, as often as every hour. For those who have not followed advice, and who have suffered painful sunburn, the main answer is to get out of the sun into the cool. Calamine lotion is probably the best local application. Great care must be taken to ensure that the blistered areas of the skin do not become infected. Anti-histamine pills by mouth are frequently helpful in cutting down the irritation and a mild sedative may well be necessary at night.

SUMMARY

Prevention of heat disorders

1 Avoid fatigue during acclimatisation.
2 Maintain your fluids. One pint per 10°F per 24 hours.
3 Maintain your salt with your fluids.
4 Never wear pure man-made fibres.
5 Be careful with the sun at first.
6 Use good quality suncreams and lotions.
7 Take two Sylvasun pills per day (but not during pregnancy) for the first two weeks. (If Sylvasun unavailable, Roavit may be substituted.)
8 For the truly sun-sensitive use a barrier cream.

6

Diseases of insanitation including travellers diarrhoea

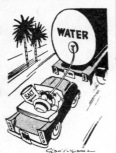

Traveller's Diarrhoea

One of the commonest and most annoying problems of overseas travel, and one which can be a great nuisance to the business executive, holiday-maker or overlander, is the frequent incidence of diarrhoea, especially in the warmer climates. Diarrhoea can be the symptom of a more serious disease but usually it is the main symptom of a condition now generally known in the medical profession as Traveller's Diarrhoea.

In the past, and to the general public, it has had many names, of which the oldest and commonest is Gippy Tummy. Men and women who served overseas in the forces in both world wars know this name only too well. In fact, it was first used by the British Army of Occupation in Egypt before the first war, and then carried on in the expanded forces of the Great War of 1914—1918. Since then, many other names have been tagged on to this complaint which is nearly always the same wherever you have it and it is only the place which differs. Going around the world eastwards, there are Basra Belly, Delhi Belly, Rangoon Runs, Hong Kong Dog, Ho Chi Minhs, Tokyo Trots, or, in Mexico, Montezuma's Revenge, Aztec Twostep, Turista. This last is perhaps the most fitting name because it is indeed the tourist who is most frequently assaulted by it.

J.E. Gordon, the eminent public health authority in the U.S.A., described it as "a notorious world-wide illness lasting one to three days, presenting often with a precipitous onset of loose stools and variable other symptoms including nausea, vomiting and abdominal cramps. It often occurs sporadically as isolated cases, though epidemics do occur within families or groups of travelers of all ages".

It may not seem to be a very serious illness, as indeed it is not, but it is annoying and exasperating. When you are making an important executive sales drive to Africa, the Far East, or even round the world, a three-day period of incapacitating diarrhoea can be a serious problem. A personal friend of mine who was the export sales director of one of Britain's largest clothing organisations brought this home to me when he told me that he was once completely 'hors de combat' during a visit to Bangkok due to traveller's diarrhoea, so that all his introductions and meetings came to naught! It could be costly to an organisation.

Similarly , those people — whatever their income — who have saved money throughout the year to give their family a holiday abroad have good reason to be upset if part of it is ruined by one or more members of the family being stricken by diarrhoea.

Equally, it spells trouble for sportsmen and sportswomen. If England's football team makes a two-week tour to several South American countries it could be an expensive and demoralising disaster if three or four members of the team cannot play because of an attack of traveller's diarrhoea. This has, in fact, occurred in the past.

It is well worthwhile to try to prevent oneself or one's family developing this diarrhoea, especially as this is possible by simple methods. Firstly, we must look at the whole problem sensibly and critically. There are so many old wives' tales about the incidence of diarrhoea that we must give real thought to the reasons for it before trying to shout preventive measures.

Looking into the problem

The man who has done more than anyone to try to answer this question is Professor B.H. Kean of Cornell University. He approached it by assessing the problem in a student community that visited Mexico City, and an exactly similar community that visited Hawaii. The diarrhoea occurred in 33 per cent of the students visiting Mexico but in only 7 per cent visiting Hawaii, although climatically there was little difference. This tends to suggest it is not just climate.

However, a Dutch naval research worker, Dr Haneveld, reporting on United Nations observers of all nationalities in the Lebanon, found the problem was far more common among those from temperate climates. In his survey he found that only 10 per cent of the Asian and South American observers had diarrhoea, compared with 40 per cent of the Europeans and North Americans.

E. Bulmer, surveying British troops in the Second World War in the Middle East, found that the longer they were overseas the less frequent the attacks, thus suggesting that some immunity against infection was developing. The United States authorities found that the annual rates of diarrhoea per thousand decreased every year a soldier served abroad; the annual rate per thousand 196, 170, 115 and 79.

Dr B. Rowe with his colleagues from the research laboratories at Colindale have carried out surveys in the Middle East and Far East and have found that at least 70 per cent of the cases of traveller's diarrhoea have been caused by infections.

To be fair, the incidence of diarrhoea among British holiday-makers in Spain, Italy and other Latin countries is so high that one wonders whether the use of olive oil in the cooking may well be acting as a laxative in addition to any infective process. Olive oil is not far removed in content from that of liquid paraffin laxative.

In addition there is the increased consumption of wine which can cause looseness and increased frequency of bowel action if not acute diarrhoea.

Further interesting facts were discovered by Professor Kean.

Firstly, he found that it occurred more in the younger adult age groups (20—30 years) than in the older groups. The older group may have travelled more and developed some immunity, or more likely they may have been more sensible over what and where they ate. He also found that 60 per cent of the cases of diarrhoea occurred in the first week that the travellers were away, and only 5 per cent after the first two weeks. Were they developing their own immunity? This is possible, but approximately one quarter had a second attack, which does not suggest developing immunity.

I was able to carry out a survey on approximately 1,200 airline ground staff members who with their wives and children had the opportunity to go on holiday on a world-wide basis because they get cheap tickets as long as there are seats unsold on the aircraft. The incidence was nearly 30 per cent in Africa, including southern Africa, 25 per cent in the Middle East, and approaching 20 per cent in southern Europe. Kean found the length of the attacks was in 57 per cent of cases one day, and in 89 per cent not more than three days. I found that 35 per cent of cases last one day, but 80 per cent not more than three days which enforces Gordon's views. Even so one to three days of illness in a tightly scheduled business trip or family holiday could cause a complete upset of arrangements.

Can this be avoided?
Going on the principle that a percentage of these cases of traveller's diarrhoea is caused by infection then surely some may be prevented by observing good food hygiene.

I must stress one final point, which is that traveller's diarrhoea is a self-limiting disease which rarely lasts longer than three days. If you develop diarrhoea which lasts for a week or more, it is not simple traveller's diarrhoea, and you must visit a doctor. Having said this one should mention the other more serious causes of diarrhoea due to insanitation and poor food hygiene.

These are far more common where the sanitary system is either initially substandard or, even if initially standard, it has been put to the extra stress which occurs when there has been a sudden and large increase in population due to tourism. Many of the popular tourist centres around the Mediterranean were little villages without drainage systems only 25 to 35 years ago, and we do not know what stresses there may be now. Even if the systems are under stress, simple preventive measures will carry you through.

The enteric group: typhoid and the paratyphoids

The most serious of the diseases of insanitation are the enteric group, typhoid, paratyphoid A, paratyphoid B and paratyphoid C. In the past in this country there were epidemics of typhoid. Just before the second world war there was one in Croydon, with several fatalities, when the water supply had become infected and, since the war, another Aberdeen epidemic caused by infected corned beef from Argentina. Nowadays, however, epidemics in the U.K. are virtually unknown, though the incidence of sporadic cases has greatly increased due entirely to overseas travel.

Paratyphoid B is an illness of Western Europe, paratyphoid A occurs in Eastern Europe and Asia, whilst paratyphoid C is practically confined to Guyana. Typhoid, which is more serious than the paratyphoids, occurs throughout the developing countries in the tropics and subtropics. It is extremely common in the Indian subcontinent and far commoner than is generally thought around the entire Mediterranean area. In 1969 there were 38 cases in one hotel in Hamamet in Tunisia, whilst in 1976 there were several cases in Spain on the Costa Brava and in 1989 on the Costa Dorada.

In 1984 there was an epidemic on the Greek holiday island of Kos where several U.K. holidaymakers developed typhoid, caused by one hotel waiter being a carrier of the typhoid organism.

All these illnesses are spread by water and milk (which has been contaminated in some way by sewage), shell fish, tinned meat, uncooked and unwashed food such as fruit, green salad, and ice creams and by the spreading of infection from lavatories to kitchens. What must be remembered is that the typhoid and paratyphoid germs are not killed by freezing, hence one must be wary of ice creams. The best way to avoid this group of diseases is to have your typhoid inoculation before you go abroad (see Chapter Two), although inoculation does not absolutely guarantee you will not develop typhoid.

Cholera

The next serious disease of insanitation is cholera, which occurs mainly in India, Pakistan, the Middle East and Africa although it has recently been reported in Peru (the first notified epidemic in the Western Hemisphere). It is a very acute diarrhoea which requires urgent and skilled medical treatment and generally occurs in epidemics which are notified to the public world wide. Any sensible person does not travel where there is an epidemic. It is spread by poor sanitation and is usually associated with poverty and overcrowding, and thus the travelling businessman or holiday-maker living in good hotels is less likely to contract it.

Bacillary dysenteries

Probably the most common of the more severe diarrhoeas are the group known as bacillary dysenteries. They are spread the same way as the enteric group by faecally-contaminated water, milk or other uncooked food, or by flies which have landed on and tainted cooked food. Acute diarrhoea usually containing blood or mucus is associated with fever, colic, abdominal pains and sometimes vomiting. A doctor should be consulted if these symptoms develop and fluids plus salts and electrolytes taken by mouth.

Salmonella infections

These infections have recently hit the headlines in the U.K. with the occurrence of salmonella-infected eggs, and are common causes of diarrhoea with fever and loss of fluids. They are particularly severe in infants and children. Typhoid is a particularly severe salmonella infection. These infections can be a particular problem with inadequately defrosted and so inadequately cooked frozen poultry.

Staphylococcal infections, brucellosis and hepatitis

Besides bacillary dysentery, other forms of diarrhoea and food poisoning can be caused by organisms, and one that is not infrequent is caused by staphylococci, the organisms which cause boils and carbuncles. This usually takes the form of a short and very sharp attack of vomiting and diarrhoea. It is frequently spread by cooks with boils or other staphylococcal infections. Milk is frequently infected by humans or cows and cream-filled cakes and other uncooked milk products can be the source of trouble. It also occurs with cold cooked food left in a warm room, or when previously cooked food is warmed up. It attacks quickly, and frequently only two to six hours after eating the infected food.

Other food or water infections are brucellosis and infective or viral hepatitis. Brucellosis is a milk-borne infection, some types of which are spread by cows' milk and some by goats' milk. All forms are particularly prevalent around the Mediterranean shores, and islands. Patients develop prolonged intermittent fever.

Infective hepatitis is sometimes known in this country as infective jaundice. It may be spread by droplet infection but certainly by faecally-infected water, salads and other uncooked foods, as the virus is known to be passed in the stools and urine. Cases have been known to occur in those who have been swimming in or near harbours where ships have emptied sewage. Infective hepatitis is an extremely common illness of overlanders to and from India and Pakistan and great care must be taken to avoid it.

This type of infective hepatitis is known as infective hepatitis A. A second form, serum hepatitis B, is more usually spread by dirty syringes or previously-used disposable syringes, body fluid and sexual intercourse. Because of this it is common in drug addicts and, hence, overlanders who are often solicited by drug traffickers, must be wary of this problem as it is a serious disease.

Campylobacter infections are similar in type and cause as salmonella infections, usually causing up to 24 hours fever before the diarrhoea starts. They have become more frequent lately.

Vibrio parahaemolyticus infections occur in the Far East from Thailand to Japan and are usually associated with shellfish.

Amoebic dysentery and Giardiasis

Amoebic dysentery is a far less acute dysentery, takes at least three weeks to develop, and symptoms may occur only after returning home. It is a milder form of diarrhoea usually without a temperature, but persistent, and associated with a general feeling of ill-health. It must be treated, or subsequent ill-health may occur, as it can infect the liver.

Giardiasis is caused by another parasite like amoebiasis and is now common amongst visitors to the Mediterranean, Middle East and Russia in particular. Unlike an amoebic infection, it remains confined to the intestines and does not spread to the liver.

How do we prevent these illnesses? There has been a persisting note of contaminated water or food in these descriptions and this therefore is where one must act.

1 *All drinking water should be boiled* and after being boiled kept in a refrigerator in clean bottles previously washed in boiled water. All ice cubes should be made of previously boiled water. The filtering of water does not purify it, only removes "bits and pieces", and it must still be boiled *after filtering* to purify it. If you boil before you filter, you B before F and you are a B.F.

The other method of purification is the use of chloramination tablets which are an absolute must for overlanders. Suitable tablets are Halozone and Sterotabs. These methods of water purification are described more fully in Appendix B.

2 *All milk should be boiled.*

3 *All cooked food should be well-cooked, recently cooked, and only once cooked.*

4 *All fruit which is not cooked and which can be peeled should be peeled — and this includes tomatoes.*

5 *Fruit which cannot be peeled and green salad such as lettuce must be sterilized by chloramination.* Salads are risky, not only because of the possibly unwashed lettuce, but also because mayonnaise is a frequent source of infection. Watercress must never be eaten in foreign parts.

6 *Do not eat food which has been cooked previously and has been left out on show* for a period, so allowing the flies to descend on it.

7 *Do not eat ice-creams or other food from unknown sources such as street hawkers.* If you want to eat an ice-cream see that it is made by one of the large proprietary firms which sell nationally. Their standards of cleanliness are likely to be far higher.

8   *Do not buy mineral waters from unknown sources:* Coca Cola and Pepsi Cola are bottled under very high standards of hygiene, and so the mineral waters made by the firms who have the local agency for "Coke" and "Pepsi" are probably the best.

9   *Do avoid fly-infested restaurants.* If the actual dining room has flies, the kitchens will have more; and a useful tip is that if the lavatories are dirty, the kitchens are likely to be dirty also.

10 Do not buy any food or drink from street hawkers.

This all seems rather long and depressing, but it is not really so. It is basic common sense and, if you follow these points, you will have a far better trip.

SUMMARY

Avoidance of diarrhoea and food poisoning.
Ten commandments.

1 Boil all drinking water and milk.

2 Be very careful of shellfish — preferably see them alive first.

3 All food well cooked and recently cooked.

4 All fruit, including tomatoes, peeled.

5 Lettuce and unpeeled fruit sterilized by chlorination — no watercress.

6 No left overs or food on display.

7 Be wary of local ice-creams — and stick to large firms.

8 Mineral waters from large firms.

9 Avoid fly-infested restaurants.

10 Do not buy any food or drink from street hawkers.

7

Further Diseases of insanitation including worm infestations

Don't eat uncooked fish or meat

Regrettably, in the warmer climates where hygiene standards are not so high, there are many forms of worm infestation. Some are spread by infested meat, fish, or water, and others by faecally-infected earth or food. In this chapter, these infestations will be discussed and also how they can easily be avoided.

Tapeworms

Everyone has heard about tapeworms although they are uncommon in developed countries. In general, most worms have what is called two hosts. Part of their life is spent living in one animal and part in another and either of the two animals may be man.

Of the four types of tapeworm, the beef tapeworm *(Taenia Saginata)* is the commonest. It leaves its eggs in the muscles of lean beef meat, and its adult life is in man where it grows to 15—20 feet. It occurs world wide although it is less common where there is adequate meat control, as in the U.K. The eggs in the beef are always killed with adequate cooking so never eat underdone or "rare" steaks in the Middle or Far East or Africa, where the meat may be infected. Steak tartare in these places is absolutely asking for trouble.

Taenia Solium is the pork tapeworm and again the egg form is in the lean pork meat. It is very rare in England and America, but does occur in Germany, India and parts of Africa. It is spread from pig to man, and can be prevented by adequate cooking. The egg form does occur in man as well as the pig, causing certain complications; but these only occur if underdone infested pork has been eaten.

The third important tapeworm is the *Taenia Echinococcus,* and here man is the host who keeps the egg form, known as the intermediate host. The egg lives in sheep, cattle and man, and the main host which houses the adult worm is the dog, but also the wolf and jackal. Man is infected by food being fouled by dog faeces, and is therefore very much a disease of insanitation, and warrants careful cooking of food. It causes a serious disease in man called hydatid disease or hydatid cyst, but it is entirely preventable. It is common where sheep are common: such as in Australia, Iceland, the sheep-rearing areas of the Middle East, particularly Cyprus which is now a tourist area, and also in the Brecon Hills of Wales.

The fourth tapeworm *Dibothriocephalus latus* occurs in man as the main host as an adult, and in pike and other fresh water fish in the egg form, but it is not very common. It is found mainly in the Haff district of the Baltic, in Finland, and in the Swiss lakes, and particularly in Lake Constance.

The answer to the beef, pork and fish tapeworms is to cook everything thoroughly.

Roundworm — Ascaris Lumbricoides

This worm has practically a world-wide distribution, but the warmer the climate, the more frequently it occurs. It is rare in the U.K. other than under insanitary conditions. With the roundworm there is no intermediate host and the human is infected by eating uncooked salads and vegetables which have been manured by human faeces, a not uncommon practice in certain communities.

Trichinella or trichiniasis

This is another small worm which infects pigs and men. It is spread by eating raw pork sausage meat and so the traveller has to be particularly careful in Germany when eating varieties of sausage meat. It has also occurred in Kenya. Fever, swelling of the eyelids and muscle pains occur with this infection.

Fishworms

In the Far East, particularly in Japan, eating raw fish is considered to be a great delicacy. This should be completely avoided as these fish are frequently infected with several types of worms which cause ill health.

Crustacea flukes

In the Far East, West Africa, and certain parts of South America, there is another worm-like parasite called a fluke which infects crayfish and crabs, and if these are eaten uncooked or undercooked, they can cause lung trouble in the human.

Hookworms

Another worm which must be mentioned, although it is not spread by infected food, is the hookworm. It lives in the duodenum in man and the eggs are passed in the stool. In underdeveloped countries and camping sites, where sanitation is bad, hookworm infection spreads easily. The egg develops in the faecally-infected soil, and the larva bores its way through the foot of the human.

This larva is a remarkably persistent and adventurous type for having penetrated the skin, it travels up through the veins into the heart. From there it passes down the lungs and then climbs up the bronchus, up the trachea or windpipe, until the latter joins with the oesophagus. When it reaches this point, it turns down again and wriggles through the oesophagus and stomach into the duodenum, to the wall of which it hooks itself. There it stays, lives on your blood and can slowly cause an anaemia. It is completely preventable so do not walk in bare feet other than on a sea-washed beach.

Avoiding worm infestations

Worms are transmitted to man through uncooked or underdone meat or fish, or through faecally contaminated food or water. Avoiding them is simple: cook all your food thoroughly, boil all your drinking water, and maintain strict hygiene when handling food and food vessels.

Schistosomiasis (also known as Bilharzia)

The final problem which I feel should be mentioned, although not strictly due to a worm, is that of schistosomiasis or bilharzia, known to the troops of both wars as "Bill Harry". This is a parasite infection which has two hosts. The primary host is man and the intermediate host is a freshwater snail. The larva develops in the snail and is then discharged into the river or lake where the snail is living. If you bathe, swim, paddle or even wash in this water the little larva will penetrate your skin. If you drink the water it will penetrate the mucous membrane of your mouth. In the human it migrates to the small blood vessels of the bladder or the rectum and intestines, depending on the type of infection. The two main types are:

Schistosomiasis Haematobium mainly attacks the bladder and causes blood in the urine. It occurs in North Africa from Morocco through to Algeria, Tunis and Egypt, in particular the Nile Valley. Running south, it occurs in northern Ethiopia, Uganda, the Congo, Zimbabwe, and South Africa, particularly Natal. In West Africa, it occurs in Liberia, Sierra Leone, and Ghana. There are also small foci in Saudi Arabia, Iran, Cyprus, southern Portugal and in Spain near Granada.

Schistosomiasis Mansoni, which causes blood-stained diarrhoea, occurs in the Nile Valley, and in a belt across Africa from Zanzibar to Sierra Leone, including all the countries of East, Central and West Africa at that level, and also occurs in Venezuela, north eastern Brazil, and the island of St Lucia in the Caribbean.

Schistosomiasis can be completely avoided by not bathing in rivers or lakes in these areas, unless you have been told categorically by the local health authority or local doctor that these rivers and lakes are free from infection. Where it is known that contact with contaminated water is likely to occur, an insect repellent should be applied to the skin beforehand. Private swimming pools may be infected if the water is drawn from a local stream, but after storage in a snail free tank for at least two days, the larva will die. Always ensure that your drinking water is boiled.

SUMMARY

Worm infestations

1 Never eat underdone or uncooked meat or fish.

2 Be very careful over shellfish: and see they are well cooked.

3 Always see your drinking water is boiled.

4 Never walk about in bare feet other than on a sea-washed beach.

5 Never bathe in rivers or lakes unless you know they are bilharzia-free.

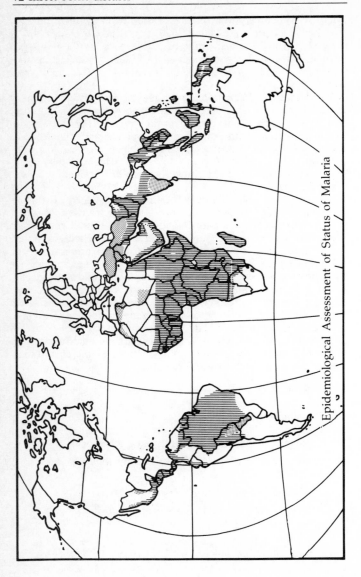

Epidemiological Assessment of Status of Malaria

8

Insect-borne diseases including malaria

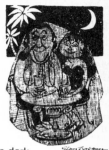

Keep well covered after dark

The second large group of diseases which occur in the warmer climates contains those that are insect-borne. With these diseases, the insect actually bites the human being, and deposits the causal organism in the patient's blood stream as distinct from the fly which picks up a small amount of faeces and deposits it on your food.

There are several of these diseases, but by far the most important is malaria.

Malaria

The first and most important thing to remember about malaria is that it can be a killer. If the more severe variety is not quickly and adequately treated it will certainly be a killer.

The second thing to remember is that it can be prevented. You need not catch malaria, if you are sensible. Remember the first point so as to ensure you follow the second point.

It is estimated that there are still over 250 million cases of malaria per annum and the death rate is about one per cent, but the death rate is higher amongst 'visiting" Europeans than in the native population which suffer repeated attacks of malaria throughout childhood. Those who survive into adult life develop an immunity which is maintained if they remain in the malarious area. They will not die of malaria but visitors from a non-malarious area have no immunity and if they receive a severe infection may die.

Those who are brought up in a malarious area, and then emigrate to a non-malarious area, in time lose a fair amount of their immunity so that when they return to a malarious area they can develop a severe attack. This is becoming quite common in Indians and Africans who have emigrated to the U.K. and then returned to their country of origin for a holiday.

Malaria is spread by the anopheline mosquito, a quite different family from the *Aedes* mosquito which spreads yellow fever.

Malaria: the background

Malaria is one of the earliest described illnesses in man. Hippocrates himself first distinguished periodic or intermittent fever, which is typical of malaria, from continuous fever. Interestingly, he further noted the connection between intermittent fever and swamp land. It was not until centuries later that it was realised that the connection was between mosquitoes breeding in swampland. But the Greeks and Romans did drain swampland for health reasons.

In 1658, Oliver Cromwell was believed to have died of malaria. It is worth noting that he was offered quinine to take, which would have cured him, but he refused on religious grounds because it was at that time known as Jesuit's Bark!

Malaria is considered to have started in Africa, and in the neolithic period crossed to Asia and Eastern Europe. In the first millennium A.D. it was taken across the Pacific to the Aztecs and Mayas in Mexico, and to the Incas in Peru. Probably in the 15th century it was taken across the Atlantic to the Caribbean by Columbus and his crew.

In this way malaria became a world-wide illness. Before eradication programmes were started it was found all over Europe as far north as 65° but now it is found scattered all over Africa, Asia, and South America. However, there are four different types with different geographical distributions.

It was in 1847 that Meckel and Frerichs first discovered that malaria was caused by a small parasite in the blood. In 1877 Manson (later Sir Patrick Manson) first showed that an insect could transfer a parasite from one man to another by biting them. This in fact was in a disease other than malaria. It was not until 1894, that Manson suggested that malaria was transmitted by mosquitoes, and it was in 1897 that Ross (later Sir Ronald Ross) showed the presence of the malaria parasite in the anopheline mosquito. It is interesting that within two years it was proved that yellow fever was transmitted by the *Aedes* mosquito in Cuba. In 1900, as with Walter Reed in Cuba, Manson transmitted malaria to volunteers who were bitten by mosquitoes in a hut in the Pontine marshes around Rome. Immediately, anti-mosquito — and in particular, larval — measures were taken in Sierra Leone, in Cuba where the Americans were still fighting a war, in Ismailia in Egypt where there were British Forces, and in Malaya.

It was in 1901 in Malaya that the first really practical move was made by the state of Selangor. The towns of Klang and Port Swettenham were to be abandoned because of the very high malaria rate. However, Malcolm Watson, the local Health Officer, constructed a drainage system that was so successful that the towns were completely rid of anopheline mosquitoes and the malaria disappeared.

Between 1904 and 1914 during the building of the Panama Canal, Gorgas and Le Prince set about ridding the area of malaria and yellow fever by eradicating first the *Aedes* and then the anopheline mosquitoes. In 1906, amongst the native workers in Panama, the malaria rate had been 821 per 1,000 men. By 1913, it had been cut down to 96 per 1,000, which is quite remarkable.

Malaria therefore occurs in any conditions which favour the presence and breeding of *Anopheles* mosquitoes. It is absent from areas free from anophelines, and as such it does not occur in the Pacific Islands east of longitude 170°E. If the temperature remains below 60°F (15.6°C), it does not occur either, even though there are anophelines around; this is because the malaria parasite needs a temperature of more than 60°F to develop. With these exceptions, malaria has been reported as far north as 65°N, as far south as 32°S, around lakes below sea level, and to an altitude of 8,500 feet, although it is rare above 6,000 feet. It occurs anywhere where it is warm and there is water.

Eradication has been tremendous since the last world war, but it is interesting that Barbados in 1927 was the first malarious area in which there was complete eradication. Obviously it was greatly helped by being an island.

One most important point in the spread of malaria is that the anopheline mosquito is an "after dark biter". So particular care must be taken not to be bitten in the evening or at night. A theoretical point is that it is the female mosquito that bites the human being whilst the males live on vegetable juices. Whether Kipling had this in mind when he wrote "The female of the species is more deadly than the male" I do not know.

Incidentally the English word "malaria" is a conversion from the French "mal-air" or bad air from the swamps, and the French name of "paludisme" is from the French word for marsh.

Malaria: the current situation

There are four different varieties of malaria but 95 per cent of all cases are one of two varieties. The more serious of these two types is *Falciparum Malaria,* sometimes known as malignant malaria, not because it has anything to do with cancer or malignant disease, but because it is so evil and can kill. It is the dominant form of malaria in tropical, West, Central and parts of East Africa. It also occurs in the Middle East, Iran, the lower end of the Arabian Gulf, parts of South, Central and Northern India, Pakistan, Bangladesh, Burma, Thailand, Malaysia, Indonesia, certain Pacific Islands, some of the West Indies, and parts of Central and South America (including Panama, Venezuela, Colombia, Brazil and inland Guyana).

The late Professor Brian Maegraith of Liverpool described it as potentially the most dangerous of all diseases that the visitor to the tropics can catch. The point about the visitor is most important because the native who has lived all his life in the malarious area has developed some immunity by repeated attacks which he has survived. The visiting European has no immunity, and is absolutely "virgin soil" for the malaria parasite. The illness develops 10—14 days after the victim is bitten by the mosquito and, so far as the patient is concerned, consists of high fever with alternate shivering and sweating, intense headache, and usually nausea or vomiting. Without treatment, the condition gets worse.

Vivax Malaria is the other main type and the two rarer types are similar to Vivax. In the non-immune visitor, the disease may be severe, but it is not dangerous to life. However, the illness will continue and recur, causing chronic ill-health, if not adequately treated.

To show how serious a problem malaria is becoming for the European traveller it is easiest to give the figures of notified cases in the U.K. There may have been even more cases which were not notified.

Malaria	Notified cases in the U.K.
1967—1970	130
1971	240
1972	363
1974	607
1975	601
1976	1162
1977	1477
1978—1990	1800-2000 in each year

Malaria has increased globally since the 1960s. In Asia, where with successful eradication, success was almost attained, *P. vivax* increased to high levels followed by *P. falciparum*. due to the spread of chloroquine resistance. From sub-Sahara the incidence of imported *P. Falciparum* has increased. Many infections were contracted in West Africa, of which a great number were in settled immigrants of the U.K. returning on home visits.

As has already been stated, malaria can and should be, prevented, but, because of the development of drug resistance in various parts of the world over the last few years, even more care and attention must be shown over the general principles because there is now no perfect drug to prevent malaria absolutely. *The maintenance of these general principles are absolutely essential.*

Prevention of malaria

Prevention of malaria can be divided into three steps:
1 Prevention of the breeding of mosquitoes.
2 If there are mosquitoes, preventing them from biting you.
3 If they bite you, preventing the malaria developing.

The first line of attack is the responsibility of the local authority and not that of the visitor, but there are minor points which can be observed by the visitor. One of the most important is not to throw out empty cans which can collect rain water and thus create breeding areas for mosquitoes. For more reasons than one, "good housekeeping" in respect of garbage and all forms of rubbish is most important.

The second line of attack is based on the principle that the anopheline mosquito bites from dusk to dawn.

● After dusk men should wear long trousers and long sleeved shirts. For women, it is a bit more difficult, but they should keep themselves as "covered" as possible.

● Use an insect repellent on the exposed skin areas. There are several of these but probably the most effective is di-ethyl toluamide which is contained in Flypel, Skee-O-Stick, Jungle Formula and Autan.

The next best are dimethylpthalate and indalone. Repellent activity usually lasts for three to four hours but this time is shortened by sweating. Some makers claim longer activity but it is safer to ignore this. Avoid eyes, lips, spectacle frames and rayon clothing.

● In a malarious area, if you are not sleeping in an air conditioned room with windows and doors shut, it is essential that you have either mosquito-proof netting over the windows which open, or a mosquito net over the bed. Even so there may be snags. With a centralised air conditioning plant which works throughout a hotel there are usually no problems but, in houses where there are usually separate air conditioning units in each room, always check that the unit fits tightly in the wall and that there are no gaps which could admit a mosquito. If there is a light on in the room and it is dark outside they will make every effort to fly in through a small gap. With window proofing and bed netting it is most essential to see there are no holes in the netting. Mosquitoes appear to be intelligent at finding their way through a net, but foolish at trying to get out. Because of these problems it is wise to have an insecticidal aerosol spray to be used in the bedroom as well. One spraying when the windows and doors are shut before dusk and another spraying before retiring to bed is a sensible precaution.

Mosquito nets and also wrist bands can be purchased which are impregnated with insect repellents.

The third line of attack is to take a tablet which will kill the malarial parasite before you develop malaria if, in effect, lines one and two have failed and you have been bitten by an infected mosquito.

Originally quinine was the drug of choice but now it is only rarely used for prophylaxis. It is interesting how war produces advances in medicine as well as surgery. In the first world war the source of quinine was cut off to the Germans so their chemists developed plasmoquine, atebrine and chloroquine. British troops, who served in Burma in the early days of the second war, will remember atebrine and how it upset them. In the second world war our source of quinine was cut off and British chemists developed proguanil or Paludrine, which is still the best prophylactic in certain areas.

D.D.T. as an insecticidal spray was originally evolved by Swiss chemists during the second world war as their potato crops were suffering from a parasitic disease, and their limited food supplies were reduced. Since then D.D.T. has become the greatest single factor in cutting down malaria on a world-wide basis.

To return to the drugs use for the prevention and treatment of malaria.

1 Proguanil — sold as Paludrine.
2 Chloroquine — sold as Avlochlor, Nivaquine, Plaquenol, Resochin, Aralen.
3 Pyrimethamine — sold as Daraprim.
4 Maloprim which is pyrimethamine and dapsone.
5 Fansidar — pyrimethamine and sulphadoxine.
6 Mefloquine.
7 Halofantrine.
8 Quinine.

Of these Fansidar and Halofantrine cannot be used for prophylaxis.

Mefloquine can only be used for prophylaxis on a short term. Quinine is only used for treatment.

In the past before the onset of drug resistance, British authorities recommended Proguanil (Paludrine), whilst most American authorities have recommended chloroquine. Personally I always recommended proguanil for several reasons:

● Whatever people may say it is easier to remember to take a tablet once a day rather than once a week, especialy as it is easy to forget which day it is if you are travelling around.
● The incubation period for malaria is ten days. If you forget a daily tablet you will probably go two days and should not suffer. If you forget a weekly tablet once, you go fourteen days between doses which could be a disaster.
● Proguanil is no good for treatment. Where there is no chloroquine resistance — chloroquine is the drug for treatment. Let us keep it for treatment.

Having said this resistance against chloroquine most regrettably has increased extensively particularly in the Far East, East Central and West Africa and South America. What is more serious is that the resistance seems to affect the serious *P. falciparum* strain. There is little resistance to proguanil. It is now considered that pyrimethamine on its own (Daraprim) is of no value at all. So from seven choices we are now down to three:

1 Proguanil.
2 Chloroquine.
3 Maloprim.

Recently the London School of Hygiene and Tropical Medicine and the Hospital for Tropical Diseases have produced new guidelines for prevention.

Area 1
Where risk is low or variable and there is no chloroquine resistance.

North Africa (Morocco, Algeria, Tunisia, Libya, Egypt).
Middle East (Turkey, Oman, Democratic Yemen, Iraq, United Arab Emirates, Saudi Arabia, Syria, Yemen).
Mauritius.
Latin America (Belize, Costa Rica, Dominican Republic, El Salvador, Guatemala, Haiti, Honduras, Mexico, Nicaragua, Paraguay, Peru, Argentina — a few areas).

In these areas Proguanil 200mgm (2 tablets) every evening or

Chloroquine as Nivaquine or Resochin (2 tablets once a week) should be taken.

Area 2
Where there is a definite risk and chloroquine resistance of varying intensity.

Asia
Afghanistan, Iran.
South Asia (Bangladesh, Bhutan, India, Nepal, Pakistan, Sri Lanka).
South East Asia (East Coast Malaysia, Thailand, China, Sarawak, Philippines, Brunei, Indonesia, Laos, Cambodia, Vietnam, Myanmar (Burma), Sabah).

Sub-Saharan Africa
Benin, Burkina Faso, Chad, Congo, Equatorial Guinea, Gabon, Ghana, Guinea, Guinea-Bissau, Cote D'Ivoire, Mali, Mauritania, Niger, Nigeria, Principe, Sao Tome, Senegal, Sierra-Leone, The Gambia, Togo.

Cameroon, Kenya, Malawi, Tanzania, Uganda, Zaire, Zambia.

Angola, Botswana, Burundi, Central African Republic, Comores, Congo, Djibouti, Ethiopia, Madagascar, Mozambique, Namibia, Rwanda, Somalia, Sudan, Swaziland, Zimbabwe, South Africa in parts of Natal and Transvaal.

Latin America
Bolivia, rural Brazil, Colombia, Ecuador, French Guinea, Guyana, Panama, Suriname, and Venezuela.

In these areas Proguanil (2 tablets) every evening and Chloroquine as Nivaquine 2 tablets once a week should be taken.

Area 3
Oceania (Papua New Guinea, Solomon Islands and Vanuata).
   Chloroquine as Nivaquine 2 tablets once a week or Proguanil 2 tablets once a day plus Maloprim one tablet once a week.

On all occasions in all these areas tablets should be started one week before arriving in the first malarial area, taken throughout the time in the areas and continued for at least four weeks after leaving the last malarial area.
   Mefloquine must not be taken for more than six weeks and need only be taken for two weeks after leaving the malarial area. It can

therefore be used for a visit of up to three weeks and started one week before. By the time this book is printed it should be available in the U.K. It is recommended for use with these limitations in the following countries: Cameroon, Kenya, Malawi, Tanzania, Uganda, Zaire, Zambia, Thailand, rural Malaysia, rural China, Indonesia, Laos, Cambodia, Vietnam, Myanmar (Burma), Philippines, Sabah.

For those perhaps out in the 'back bush' and away from prompt medical treatment in a highly malarial area who develop a fever, immediate emergency treatment should be taken in the form of Fansidar 3 tablets together ONCE or Mefloquine 3 tablets ONCE. However if Mefloquine is being used for prophylaxis Fansidar must be used for treatment.

A few points to add:

1 Malaria is one of the infections that pass across the placental barrier to infect the foetus. It is therefore absolutely essential to take anti-malarials in pregnancy but they should be limited to proguanil and/or chloroquine.

2 For long-term residents chloroquine must not be taken for more than five years, for if continued it can cause eye problems. It is also contra-indicated in people who have psoriasis, a skin disorder.

3 The dose of one tablet per week of Maloprim must not be exceeded.

4 Proguanil has no serious side effects, which is another point in its favour, but occasionally mouth ulcers occur, which are commoner when it is taken in conjunction with chloroquine.

5 The dosage plan for children is as follows:

Age	Weight	Chloroquine Proguanil	Maloprim
0 — 5 weeks		⅛ Adult dose	Not recommended
6 weeks—5 months		¼ Adult dose	⅛ Adult dose
6 — 11 months		¼ Adult dose	¼ Adult dose
1 — 5 years	5—19 kg	½ Adult dose	½ Adult dose
6 — 11 years	20—39 kg	¾ Adult dose	¾ Adult dose
12 years upwards		Adult dose	Adult dose

Nivaquine (Chloroquine) is put up in a syrup for children. The recommended doseage is as follows:

1 — 2 years	1 x 5ml teaspoon
3 — 4 years	1½ x 5ml teaspoon
5 — 7 years	2 x 5ml teaspoon

    8 — 10 years   3 x 5ml teaspoon
    11 — 12 years   4 x 5ml teaspoon

To summarise:

1 Malaria can kill.
2 Being bitten by the anopheline mosquito can usually be
   prevented by taking sensible precautions.
   (a) Keep yourself well-covered with clothing after dark.
   (b) See you have good mosquito proofing on the windows of
   your living quarters and bedrooms or mosquito netting around
   beds if you are not in a centrally air-conditioned house.
   (c) Use an aerosol insecticidal spray at dusk in your living
   quarters and at dusk and bed time in your bedrooms.
   (d) Use an insect repellent on your skin. Wrist and ankle bands
   impregnated with insect repellent can now be purchased.
3 Malaria can usually be prevented by taking anti-malarial
   prophylactic tablets as set out in the regime already stated, but
   the general precautions in 1 and 2 above are absolutely essential.

A great deal of work is being done on anti-malarial vaccines but it
is a complicated process and success is still a long way off.

For a traveller who develops a severe fever in a malarial area, and
who is away from prompt medical attention, emergency treatment
should be considered.

Either **one dose** of 3 tablets of Fansidar or **one dose** of 3 tablets
of Mefloquine is the answer. However Mefloquine must not be used
if it is already being taken for prophylaxis.

These are interim emergency measures and medical advice must
still be sought without delay.

The chloroquine resistant areas are shown in the table.

Malaria is by far the most important of the insect-borne diseases,
but there are others which must be considered.

Filariasis

This is a tropical illness and not to be confused with malaria. It
takes three different forms each of which is spread by a different
insect. One form which causes inflammation of the lymphatic
glands is spread by mosquitoes. Initially it looks like the tender red

Chloroquine resistant areas

Africa

Angola
Benin
Botswana
Burkino Faso
Burundi
Cameroon
Central Africa Republic
Chad
Comores
Congo
Djibouti
Equatorial Guinea
Ethiopia
Gabon
Gambia
Ghana
Guinea
Guinea-Bissau
Ivory Coast
Kenya
Liberia
Madagascar
Malawi
Mali
Mauritania
Mozambique
Namibia
Niger
Nigeria
Rwanda
Sao Tome & Principe
Senegal
Sierra Leone
Somalia
South Africa
Sudan
Swaziland
Tanzania
Togo
Uganda
Zaire
Zambia
Zimbabwe

Asia

Bangladesh
Burma
India
Indonesia
Kampuchea
Laos
Malaysia
Nepal
Pakistan
Papua New Guinea
Philippines
Sri Lanka
Thailand
Vanuata
Vietnam

South America

Bolivia
Brazil
Colombia
Ecuador
French Guiana
Guyana
Suriname
Venezuela

line of lymphangitis which may run up the arm with a poisoned finger. If filariasis is untreated it may subsequently cause elephantiasis.

The two other forms affect the eye. One is spread by certain forest flies (Chrysops) and the other by the buffalo gnat or Simulium. All three infections are more likely to be caught by agricultural workers or those on construction sites — particularly dams because the insects like water — than by visitors. It is rare for town dwellers to catch them, but once more the infection is prevented by the use of mosquito netting, insect repellents, and insecticidal sprays.

Kala Azar

This is a debilitating infection with a long-term fever. It is spread by the sandfly which regrettably is so small that no mosquito net can keep it out. A "sandfly net" would not allow enough air and thus it is another reason for using a repellent. Besides occurring in scattered areas of India, West, Central and East Africa, it also occurs in circumscribed areas of the Mediterranean shores, especially where holiday-makers go. In particular, the Mediterranean variety tends to attack children. Areas of risk are southern Greece and the Greek Islands; parts of the coast of Yugoslavia; the toe of Italy; Sicily; the western end of the French Riviera; Corsica; parts of the western and souther coastline of Spain; and the southern tip of Portugal — all ever-popular resorts of the European inclusive-tour holiday-maker.

Sandfly fever and dengue fever

These are two other insect-borne infections, both more unpleasant than serious in that they are like a severe flu. Dengue is also known as "Breakbone Fever", due to the intense limb-ache and backache. The first is naturally spread by the sandfly, and the second by the *Aedes* mosquito. Both occur in the eastern Mediterranean, sub-tropics and tropics. Avoid them by using mosquito-netting and, most important, insect repellent.

Finally, two illnesses spread by insects must be mentioned if only to reassure:

Yellow fever

If you have been inoculated against yellow fever within the last ten years, you will not get it.

Sleeping sickness or trypanosomiasis

This is a serious illness, but due to intense work carried out in West, Central and East Africa to control the tsetse fly which spreads it, the areas where it occurs are now limited. One variety occurs in the Gambia, Sierra Leone, Ghana, Nigeria and Cameroon; and the other in Zimbabwe and East Africa. Here again it is the person living or working in the rural areas, plus the game park visitor on "safari" holidays, who is affected, not the town-dweller.

SUMMARY

Insect-borne diseases including malaria

1 Keep yourself well covered after dark.
2 See you have good mosquito proofing either on the window or over the bed.
3 Use an insect repellent on your skin — frequently.
4 Use an insecticidal spray in your bedroom.
5 Take your anti-malarial for at least one week before entering the first malarious area until four weeks after leaving the last.

Lassa fever

Although not insect-borne this is perhaps an appropriate place to mention Lassa fever as it has been regrettably much publicised by the media. This recently described disease occurs in Nigeria, Sierra Leone, Liberia and probably the Central African Republic and is not known to occur elsewhere. Although it is an unpleasant illness with probably a 50 per cent mortality rate, there has been only one known second generation case developing outside Africa, and that was in a laboratory technician who had mishandled infected blood. Thus much of the drama concerning its spread is probably unnecessary. Regrettably this is due to the media. After three cases were treated at the Hospital for Tropical Diseases in London, 908 contacts were traced, several of them close contacts, and none developed lassa fever.

9

Direct contact diseases including those from domestic animals bites and stings

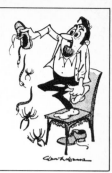

Tuberculosis

In the developed countries this usually takes the form of tuberculosis of the lungs, but in the tropics it appears in many different forms, and is a far more acute disease. Tuberculosis, and the spread of it, is encouraged by overcrowding, poverty, poor nutrition, lack of personal hygiene, and the tropical climate. As such, it can be rampant in the poorer areas of the townships.

It is obviously of no concern to the holiday-maker or the businessman making a quick trip to the tropics and back, but it should be of great concern to the person who is going out to work with the native poor. This applies in particular to our own young school-leavers or university graduates, who have joined Voluntary Service Overseas for one or two years to help in the teaching and training of young people in the developing countries and also to the American counterpart, the Peace Corps. These volunteers do great work, but they will be far more bother than they are worth, both to themselves and everyone else, if they go down with tuberculosis.

Those who are going to work amongst the poor in developing countries should be immunised against tuberculosis if they have not already had an attack of apparent or non-apparent tuberculosis. The procedure is to arrange through your own doctor for a specific skin test to be carried out, the result of which shows whether you have had tuberculosis or not.

If, following the test, it is suggestive, because of a negative result, that you have never had any tuberculosis infection and are therefore likely to develop one if you are in contact with tuberculosis, arrangements should then be made for you to have a B.C.G. inoculation against tuberculosis before travelling abroad. There is no conclusive evidence how long this inoculation lasts, but it is, almost certainly, at least five years.

Besides the voluntary workers such as V.S.O. and the Peace Corps, "overlanders" to and from India and Pakistan and through South America live rough at times and mix with the local inhabitants.

If you have been given a B.C.G. immunisation against tuberculosis you should not have any further immunisations IN THE SAME ARM for at least three months.

Leprosy

In a number of ways this disease is rather akin to tuberculosis, but it is a chronic condition, and only acquired by prolonged close contact with leprous patients, and then usually only by children. Leprosy appears through history and of course it is often quoted in the Bible as a foul infectious disease. As a result, many people going to the tropics are in fear of developing leprosy but it is not highly infectious. Equatorial Africa is its most common site, with a moderate incidence in India, Sudan, Ethiopia, Angola and the northern part of South America. For the average traveller, including people staying a year or two in these parts, the risk can be dismissed.

Sexually transmitted diseases

The third group of direct contact diseases are the sexually transmitted diseases which understandably occur in all countries. Just because a country is underdeveloped, there is no reason to support that sexual transmitted diseases have not developed there. I am afraid some wishful thinkers are under this impression and usually change their views through bitter experience!

What is particularly worrying is that in many places around the world resistance has developed to all the common antibiotics used in the treatment of these diseases. This presents a terrible problem and makes it all the more important that the traveller does not render himself vulnerable.

AIDS, or to give it its full name Acquired Immuno-deficiency Syndrome, is a world wide disease carried by the H.I.V. virus which can break down the body's immune or defence system and so lead to fatal infections and some forms of cancer. The infection may be dormant for years and although the patients are infectious they may not develop symptoms for a long time. Due to the breakdown of the immune or defence system patients may develop serious disease when a normal person would be able to cope satisfactorily with the infection. An infection of the lungs known as pneumo-cystis carinii pneumonia is particularly serious with AIDS patients.

Kaposi's sarcoma, a rare form of cancer, usually of the skin, but which can effect other parts of the body, is far commoner in AIDS patients. AIDS is spread mainly by sexual contact. The virus can be transmitted from any person to his or her sexual partner (man to woman, vice versa and man to man or woman to woman). It is also spread by contaminated blood transfusions, used needles or any skin piercing instruments (tattooing, ear piercing, acupuncture). An infected mother can transmit it to her child during or shortly after birth. It is not spread by casual or working contact, insects or insect bites, swimming pools, public transport, food, water, air, lavatories, eating utensils, laundry, coughing or sneezing.

Do not have sex with prostitutes — male or female, or casual acquaintances. It is claimed that all prostitutes in Mombasa have AIDS. You cannot tell by appearances and he or she can look healthy.

If you insist on sexual contact men should wear a condom from start to finish and women should insist that the man wears one.

Vaginal, anal and oral sex can spread AIDS, but reducing the number of partners will lower the risk.

What about blood transfusions? Many countries report that they are screening blood for AIDS. If a blood transfusion is needed you and your close relatives should insist that only screened blood is used. It is essential that everyone who travels or lives overseas — and sensible to try and persuade your relatives, friends and companions — to know their own blood group. It may then be possible that, if one of the group needs a blood transfusion, someone else in the group may be able to provide the necessary blood.

Avoid injections if possible, and if you have an injection make sure the syringe and needle come from a sterile package. Travellers can purchase suitable packs of syringe, needles and stitching material to take with them from places like M.A.S.T.A. at the London School of Hygiene and Tropical Medicine, British Airways Immunisation Centre and Trailfinders Medical Advisory and Immunisation Centre but make sure you have a covering letter signed by a doctor that this is purely for medical use by a physician.

If you do have sex with a prostitute or casual contact whilst abroad, seek advice from a specialist in sexually transmitted diseases on return home before having sex with your normal partner.

Certain countries demand a certificate of clearance that a prospective long term resident has not been infected with the AIDS virus.

Iraq demands it of all entrants. There blood is tested on arrival and foreign certificates are not accepted, unless approved by the Iraqi consulate in the country of departure.

The U.S.A. demands it of prospective immigrants, whilst Kuwait, Papua New Guinea and Saudi Arabia demand a certificate that the applicant is H.I.V. negative before granting a work permit.

Belgium, Finland, Germany and India demand it from foreign students intending to study in their countries.

China and the Philippines want certificates from those applying for more than one year's residence.

India also requires it from tourists staying for more than one month.

The highest prevalence of AIDS is in the Congo, where there are 60 cases per 100,000 of population; and next the U.S.A. with approximately 30 per 100,000. Of the next nine countries with decreasing frequency of cases seven are from Sub-Sahara Africa and the other two are Haiti and the Dominican Republic. By 31 March 1989 at the W.H.O. collaborating centre on AIDS 21,857 AIDS cases had been reported by 31 countries in the European region. The number of reported cases had increased by 79 per cent since March 1988 and of those 87.4 per cent were males and 42 per cent belonged to the 25—34 years age group; 51.3 per cent were homosexuals or bi-sexuals, 27.5 per cent were intravenous (I.V.) drug users and 7.7 per cent were infected by heterosexual contact. In women 55.7 per cent of cases were intravenous (I.V.) drug users.

The number of cases in the I.V. drug group continues to rise at a considerable rate. In one year there has been an increase of 130.6 per cent among I.V. drug users compared with 60.8 per cent amongst homo/bisexual men. This increase is particularly evident in Italy and Spain. Trends in prevalence made per million population suggest the start of a levelling off in northern European countries which is not apparent in other countries. During the next decade AIDS prevention and control programmes are projected to be potentially capable of preventing almost half of the new HIV infections which may occur between 1988 and the 2000. On the other hand more than half of the approximate five million AIDS cases which are projected for the next decade will occur regardless of how effective the HIV/AIDS prevention efforts may be, since the AIDS cases will be developing in those infected with HIV before

1989. Up to the end of the 1980s, it is estimated that fewer than one million AIDS cases will have occurred, and during the 1990s several million AIDS cases will develop.

Rabies

Of all the diseases transmitted from domestic animals to man rabies is by far the most terrible. Other than the 1970 scare in Camberley when a dog was found to have the disease (which is transmitted from dog to man), and three cases in the U.K. in the last 14 years, an overlander from India and one in a veterinarian from West Africa in 1976, and one in 1981 in a lady from Gloucestershire who had been on holiday in India, rabies has been stamped out entirely in Britain. This is because of the insistence that all dogs when they are brought into this country from abroad have to spend six months in quarantine. This is absolutely right because if rabies is ever allowed to develop, it is always fatal. Rabies is unknown in Australia because they have the same strict quarantine rules as in Britain, but is found in Germany, and is fairly common in France, Russia and the U.S.A.

It is common in the Indian sub-continent, Thailand and the Philippines and also in parts of South America. In Latin America, Trinidad and Jamaica it is spread by vampire bats while in the U.S.A. it is spread by the grey squirrel, and in Canada by the fox and the wolf. Although dogs are the most important carrier of rabies worldwide, cats, foxes, skunks, mongooses and deer can also be infected. What also must be remembered is that any animal may be bitten by a rabid animal so in a rabid country any animal could have rabies so *any excited* animal can be a cause for worry.

What also is a matter of concern is that rabies is spreading across Western Europe in a westerly direction at an alarming rate, such that it may soon reach the channel ports, which will make quarantine even more important. With the advent of the Channel Tunnel supervision will have to be extremely strict.

The rabies virus usually enter the human through 'broken skin' caused by the bite of a rabid dog; but if there is a scratch, cut or other break in the skin, then the infection can be spread by the dog licking that break as the virus is in the animal's saliva. However, the virus can also penetrate unbroken mucous membranes such as the linings of the mouth and nose or the covering of the eyes.

The name rabies comes from the Latin *rabere* to rave, and the dog is typically wild and uncontrolled.

Immediately someone has been bitten by what might be a rabid dog the wound should be washed thoroughly with copious amounts of soapy water or detergent, and water poured into the wound. If possible, the wound should be put under a tap turned on full so that most of the saliva containing the virus may be washed away. Do not scrub the wound for this may push the infection in deeper. After washing under a running tap for at least five minutes apply an antiseptic such as tincture of iodine or 40—70% alcohol but whisky, gin or vodka can be used as they contain over 40% alcohol. Having satisfactorily cleaned the wound, the patient must then go immediately to a local physician who will arrange for anti-rabietic serum and a vaccine to be given. He may give it himself or more likely he may refer the patient to hospital as the necessary treatment can usually only be obtained at a major medical centre.

The incubation period for the development of rabies is usually 30 — 60 days but it has been known to be as little as four days and as long as two years. It depends on the extent of the bite. The time is shorter if bitten on the shoulder than if bitten on the foot as the infection passes up the nerves to the brain. On no account should medical attention be delayed until the patient has returned to his or her country. The new vaccine is effective, safe and without side effects and consists of an initial immediate injection with repeats on the third, seventh and fourteenth days. Serum is applied to the wound on the first visit. The older unpleasant vaccine which was given into the abdominal wall on 21 consecutive days is no longer used.

Immediate cleaning of the wound, combined with follow up treatment with vaccine and serum is successful in preventing the development. One must repeat that pre-exposure prophylactic vaccination against rabies (described in Chapter Two) just gives more time to get post-exposure treatment but *is not sufficient in itslef when someone is bitten.*

Tick typhus

There are two other illnesses which may be carried by the domestic dog. The hard-backed ticks which sometimes inhabit the coats of dogs in the tropics (especially if they are long-haired) may carry the germ of tick typhus fever which occurs mainly in Ethiopia, East Africa and South Africa. It is like an extremely severe influenza and can be fatal. The tick can move direct from dog to man, or from dog to long grass to man, and this is another good reason why you should not walk about unshod or badly shod in "flip-flops" as you may be bitten on the foot by a tick. It is also a good reason to ensure that your dog, if you have one, is kept clean and frequently "de-ticked".

Other infections from domestic animals

The third point with domestic dogs is that in the last ten years it has been realised that a common worm infection can infect man and can cause eye disease. A dog worm infection is more common in the tropics than in temperate climates and so frequent "de-worming" of dogs is essential.

It is reckoned that in Calcutta 80 per cent of dogs are infected with *Toxocara canis,* 37 per cent in Ibadan, Nigeria and 28 per cent in Dar-es-Salaam, Tanzania. Even in London 12.8 per cent of 1,000 stool specimens from dogs were infected.

The infections spread by cows, goats and pigs, have already been discussed under diseases of insanitation and include from unboiled milk — typhoid, dysentery, poliomyelitis and brucellosis — and the worm infections spread by underdone meat.

I will turn next to the troubles caused by direct contact: namely bites and stings.

Snakebites

The first principle to be remembered with snakes is that in general they do not attack for the pleasure of it but only in self defence: if disturbed, trodden on or cornered when they cannot escape. They usually hunt at night and dislike the light so when you are walking in the dark, shine a torch in front of you, and they will usually scuttle away. When a snake gets into a house, it usually hides in a dark corner. Frequently small ones will hide in a shoe so always shake a shoe before putting it on.

Travellers rarely suffer from snakebites and it is usually members of the local rural tribes, especially children, who are bitten. It is useful to know whether there are snakes in the areas where you are travelling and which varieties are there, but it is not a matter of taking anti-venom with you as it has to be kept cool. Rely on local medical services to provide the correct anti-venom — which should only be used if there are definite signs of generalised poisoning.

The most important thing about bites by poisonous snakes is that more than one half of the victims will have minimal or no poisoning. Only around 25 per cent will develop generalised poisoning. *Hence one must remember that a poisonous snakebite does not necessarily mean snakebite poisoning.*

It must be admitted that a snakebite, whether the snake is poisonous or not, can be very frightening.

First aid treatment given by the victim or his friends before the arrival of the doctor must be simple.

1. First, bearing in mind the small number who are adversely affected is a matter of reassurance, which is statistically truthful and medically helpful. Even the most poisonous, such as cobras, frequently do not inject enough venom to be harmful. The speed of death from snakebites, even when there is poisoning, has been greatly exaggerated. With cobras and mambas it is usually hours and with vipers days, which means that there is nearly always time for successful treatment.

2. Wipe the site of the bite and cover it with a clean cloth.

3. Immobilize the limb with a splint and arrange for transfer to a doctor or hospital if available.

4. DO NOT apply a tourniquet unless you know the bite is from a snake whose venom contains a nerve poison such as cobras, mambas and wraits amongst others. If you do, apply it firmly but not tightly and release it every thirty minutes or gangrene may occur. The tourniquet should be applied just above the bite on the limb affected.

5. DO NOT incise the wound as it could then become infected.

6. DO NOT suck the wound.

7. DO NOT apply potassium permanganate crystals.

8. Give paracetamol (Panadol) for pain. DO NOT give aspirin as it may cause bleeding from the stomach.

9. If the snake has been killed, but only if it is well and truly dead, lift it up by its tail and take it to the hospital. It will help the doctor to give the correct anti-venom.

Lizards are non-poisonous except for one variety living in the deserts of Mexico and Arizona, so they can be dismissed as of no concern.

Scorpions are a problem in the tropics and are common in Africa, Central and South America and the Caribbean but less frequent in Asia. Resembling a beetle and about two inches long, with a slightly larger tail, the scorpion is nocturnal in habit and spends the day hiding under stones, or, like the small snake, in shoes. Once again, they attack only when disturbed, but if you put your shoe on a scorpion would consider it was being molested. The sting is in the tail but a scorpion has claws in front which grip you, then swings its tail over its head and pumps in the poison.

The sting is like a severe bee or wasp sting and there may be generalised symptoms such as muscular cramps, sweating, fever and vomiting, but this is usually confined to children. It has been found that the local pain is frequently relieved by injection of a local anaesthetic so it is worthwhile visiting a doctor or hospital.

Spiders Nearly all have poison glands but the poison is intended to kill insects and a bite from the majority of spiders is minimal, and may even go unnoticed. There are only a few spiders which are dangerous and, even with these, the symptoms disappear in a few days. The spiders in this group are the redbacked spiders of Australia and New Zealand, and the notorious Black Widow. Deaths are unusual but may occur in children. Anti-venoms are available in the countries where there are these dangerous spiders.

Bees and wasps in the U.K. and, in warmer climates, ants and centipedes can also sting. Ammonia, if available, is probably the best treatment to put on all these stings, and calamine lotion will always give some relief.

The problem here is that if someone is stung frequently a hypersensitivity may develop which shows itself by increasing local reactions to stings. If the hypersensitivity gets worse there may be general reaction consistent which an acute allergy with bronchial asthma, when urgent medical attention is required.

Ants, beetles, caterpillars and centipedes can all cause local pain and sometimes blistering.

Leeches, with their blood-sucking habits, will be found only in rivers or marshy areas. They will never bite if you use an insect repellent so, when in this type of terrain, put the repellent on your legs and socks as well as on your face and hands. If you are bitten by a leech it hangs on but you must not try to pull it off or it will leave its claws inside. Apply salt, vinegar, the lighted end of a cigarette, or a needle to the leech to make it drop off. To the bite apply an antiseptic cream.

The **chigoe flea, chigger or jigger,** is a flea found in Africa, the West Indies, and North and South America. It lives in dry, sandy soil, dust and ashes and also in badly-kept quarters, stables and, particularly, poultry pens. It is common around the edge of sandy beaches; but not on sand that is sea-washed.

It is the female chigger which is the main trouble in that, when she has been fertilised by the male, she burrows into the skin of the nearest warm-blooded animal she can find, nearly always in the foot. There in the warmth she ovulates and gradually grows to the size of a small pea. As a result, there is much local irritation and the area usually becomes infected. The eggs are laid, and the skin above and around ulcerates, leaving an infected sore. The best treatment is to use a sterilised needle to remove the insect entirely before the ulceration occurs, and apply antiseptic ointment. A very good reason again for not walking about barefoot.

The **tumbu fly** is another egg-laying fly which inhabits East, Central and West Africa south of the Sahara. In its life cycle the female fly lays her eggs on dry sand and soil which has been contaminated by the excreta of animals, particularly rodents and man. The larvae which hatch can live for a week or two in the soil until they become attached to a passing or resting host.

In Africa it is very common for the domestic staff to lay out the washing on dry soil to dry in the sun and fresh air. This is one of the commonest causes of the spread of the larvae of the tumbu fly. The larvae climb on to the shirt, vest, pants or any other nether garment, from which they burrow just under the skin leaving their posterior breathing openings on a level with the skin. Usually multiple boil-like lumps appear. Treatment is to put liquid paraffin on the lumps and after a few applications they can usually be squeezed out.

Jellyfish poisoning is an unpleasant form of sting which occurs in sea-bathing. Like the human being, the jellyfish family prefers warm to cold seas and, as such, they are far more common in the Mediterranean and Indian Ocean than in the North Sea or English Channel. Although the actual fish is like a large flat colourless jelly there is one long delicate process coming out from the surface known as the trigger hair. When this is touched, the hair everts and several sharp barbs sting the human. The Portuguese Man-o'-War is a particularly unpleasant type of jellyfish, with many tentacles, and is tinged bluish purple in colour. They frequently swim around in shoals and, if they are present it is advisable not to enter the water.

A jellyfish sting can be extremely painful, causing acute shock, which may lead to collapse in the water with serious results. Morphia is sometimes necessary for the pain. Subsequently, soothing lotions, such as calamine, should be applied locally and antihistamine pills taken by mouth. Fever may ensue, following the sting, and medical advice should be sought.

Sea anemones sting in a similar manner to jellyfish, but usually over a smaller area, and to a milder extent with not such serious results. Treatment is the same.

Sting rays, weevil fish and other poisonous fish may lie in the sand and they can sting if you walk on them. The sting and treatment is similar to the jellyfish.

Sea snakes are found from the Arabian Gulf to southern Japan in the Indian Ocean and the Pacific Ocean: and also off the northern tropical shores of Australia. They can be recognised from their flat rudder-like tail unlike the harmless water snake that has a round, tapering tail. These sea snakes are highly poisonous, but they do not inhabit shallow water and their victims are usually local offshore fishermen. Inshore bathers and paddlers are rarely affected.

SUMMARY

Direct contact diseases, including those from domestic animals, bites and stings

1 If you are bitten by an excited dog, wash the bite thoroughly and go at once to a doctor or hospital.

2 If you keep a dog in the tropics, de-flea and de-worm it regularly and have it vaccinated against rabies.

3 In a snake area always take a torch out at night. Tuck your trousers tight round your ankles.

4 Always shake a shoe before putting it on.

5 Do not walk around barefooted.

6 With a snakebite, reassure the patient and clean the wound. Do not incise. Go to the hospital. Only apply a tourniquet if you *know* the bite is from a cobra, mamba or krait — and then not too tight.

Stonefish are found on the shores of the islands of the Indian Ocean such as the Seychelles, around the Malaysian coasts and further east to Indonesia and New Guinea. They look like a stone, as their name suggests and if bathers around a coral reef walk on them a poison is injected into the feet. There is usually severe and immediate pain accompanied frequently by severe shock. First aid treatment involves bathing the foot in water as hot as is bearable or an Epsom Salts solution, but a doctor's advice should be sought as other help can be given.

Certain fish and shellfish if eaten can cause symptoms of paralysis associated with diarrhoea and vomiting within a matter of hours. They are puffer fish, barracuda, tuna and mackerel. Vomiting and bowel movement should be encouraged with emetics and aperients. If the symptoms are mild antihistamines may be sufficient but, if there is acute bronchial spasm, adrenaline may be necessary. Rarely the breathing muscles may be paralysed and then a ventilator may be necessary.

10

Special for overlanders

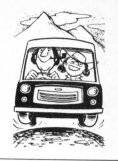

"Overlanding" is a form of travel which has increased many times over during the last 10 to 15 years. The most popular routes are from Europe to the Indian subcontinent, and across Africa, but some venture as far as South East Asia. Many from Australia and New Zealand do a "one way trip" either on their way to Europe or on their way home. Another popular route in the last few years has been across the northern part of South America.

The great benefits of travelling overland are the ability to see the countries as they really are — and by this one means seeing the lands as they really are — and travel in an economical manner. Whether one travels by bus, Land-Rover or car, whether it is all arranged beforehand or done on a hitch-hiking basis, overlanding offers tremendous experiences for everyone and great companionship.

However, overlanding definitely has its problems, not least of which are the medical aspects of the journey. Before discussing the medical side of this way of travelling one must mention a serious aspect which although not truly medical can have serious medical implications.

A warning

Regrettably, a fair percentage of overlanders are already taking drugs in some form or another before they start their journey, whether of soft or hard variety. During the journey to India they pass through areas, in particular Afghanistan, where all these drugs are sold by hard core traffickers. Obviously those who are already on drugs will find the traffickers and purchase further supplies. What is the great worry is that the traffickers will search out those who are not already taking drugs and, by one means or another, will persuade many to purchase their wares so that many overlanders who left Europe not taking drugs arrive back home as established drug takers. I have known patients and others who have been pressurised by this 'sales talk'. Some have resisted it but others have succumbed and thus have started taking addictive drugs purely as a result of participating in an absolutely innocent overland trip. *This is something about which every overlander should be wary.* There is the added worry that, when they are returning home some overlanders travel through Iran or southern Russia, where the laws against drug smuggling are strict and the penalties heavy, including the death sentence.

Preventive measures

To return to the truly medical aspects of these trips. By the very nature of the exercise a percentage of the living must be rough and thus, before setting off on the journey, every form of preventive inoculation must be seriously considered.

Inoculation: check list for overlanders
All possible inoculations must be carried out well before travel.

● **Smallpox,** has been eradicated and vaccination against it is no longer necessary.

● **Yellow fever** vaccination is not required for overlanders in Asia in either direction but, for those carrying out a similar trip in the northern part of South America or Central Africa, it is essential.

● **Cholera** vaccination is demanded by some of the Asian and African countries through which this type of traveller is passing, and is advisable.
Once more one must stress that the following vaccinations are by far the most important from the traveller's health point of view.

● **Typhoid** vaccinations are absolutely essential for all overlanders. The type of country through which they are passing has a high incidence of typhoid and on many occasions they will be eating under unhygienic conditions, as a result of which they could easily develop typhoid fever.

● **Tetanus.** All overlanders must be fully protected against tetanus. If for any reason they suffer an accident or injury in which the skin is broken it is unlikely for them to be near satisfactory hospital facilities at the time. The likelihood of contracting tetanus is always present and they must take every precaution to prevent it by being fully protected through inoculation.

● **Poliomyelitis** vaccination is essential. For fear of being accused of repetition one must remind travellers that poliomyelitis is primarily a disease of warm climates and it is still rampant in the developing countries where poliomyelitis immunisation is not practised. As such it is advisable for overlanders to have a full course of vaccination if their last course was more than five years previously.

● **Gamma globulin** for Hepatitis A is also essential. It is proven to be extremely effective in the prevention of infective hepatitis A provided the time limitation of its effectiveness is remembered. Most companies running overland groups demand that their clients are immunised with gamma globulin.

● **Plague.** Vaccination is only necessary for visitors to upland areas of Africa and South America and it is therefore not required for those going through Asia. It can have a severe reaction and must not be given with other vaccinations.

● **Rabies.** In view of the environmental circumstances to which overlanders are subjected one must seriously consider rabies inoculation. If bitten by a rabid, or possibly rabid, animal immediate treatment is necessary and, if "overlanding", this could well not be possible. Hence, prophylactic inoculation is strongly advised. It consists of two injections four weeks apart. If continued prophylaxis is required then a third dose should be given 6-12 months later and boosters every 2-3 years.

● **Meningococcal meningitis.** This is essential for overlanders in Africa and Asia as they pass through the established meningococcal meningitis areas — namely sub-Saharan Africa and northern India and Nepal.

● **Hepatitis B.** It would be sensible for overlanders to be immunised against Hepatitis B with Engerix B because their trips last several months and they pass through areas where medical facilities are poor and sterile syringes and needles may not be available.

● **B.C.G.** is the last inoculation to be considered. B.C.G. is the antituberculosis inoculation named after the French physicians who worked out the principal of antituberculosis inoculation, Bacille Calmette-Guerin. Tuberculosis in various forms affecting lungs, bones, joints, the abdomen and other parts of the body, is common amongst the poorer communities in the developing countries, especially in India, Pakistan, Afghanistan and surrounding countries. As such, overlanders who will be mixing with these communities should be adequately protected.

Before having B.C.G. vaccination, the recipient should have a Mantoux skin test which shows whether the recipient has an immunity to tuberculosis due to a previous conquered infection or whether there is no immunity and a liability to catch tuberculosis if in contact with an active infection. If the Mantoux test shows the latter then it is essential to have a B.C.G. vaccination. This type of vaccination can cause a rather trying ulcer which is slow to heal and it should be carried out well before the time of intended travel.

No live vaccine must be given within three weeks of B.C.G. and no other vaccinations in the B.C.G. arm for three months.

Intestinal infections

The commonest problems to assault overlanders are intestinal infections. Travelling as they do, they must live rough on occasions and the chances of developing one or more intestinal infections are high.

One of the commonest ways in which they pick up an infection or a parasitic infestation is through unsatisfactory water. The best way of purifying water is adequate boiling but this is not always possible and it is therefore essential for overlanders to take with them an adequate supply of water sterilising tablets. There are several varieties which can be purchased from any pharmacy but Halozone, Sterotabs and Chloramine tablets are satisfactory. Tincture of iodine can also be used as mentioned in Appendix B.

The main principles concerning the avoidance of intestinal infections have been clearly laid down in Chapter Six and these principles are even more important. For overlanders all food should be well and recently cooked and uncooked food should be avoided.

Malaria

Although the commonest problems may be the intestinal infections, the most serious so far as immediate life or death is concerned is obviously malaria. Whether it is the Asian, African or the South American trail, the traveller is entering a malarious area. It has been clearly written in Chapter Eight that malaria can kill and can kill fairly rapidly. Overlanders are frequently a long way from adequate medical treatment. Once a severe attack of malaria has been established the patient can die within a week unless a high standard of medical attention is available. Hence it is absolutely essential that an antimalarial prophylactic is taken on a regular basis, and once more it must be reiterated that proguanil (Paludrine) on a daily basis is by far the best on the Middle East trail. For South America, India and Nepal two tablets of chloroquine once a week should be added.

As well as taking prophylactic tablets it is essential to have personal mosquito nets if camping out or living in quarters which are unlikely to be mosquito proofed. (Preferably of 50 denier terylene filament yarn, 20—24 threads to the inch.) An adequate supply of insect repellents and insecticidal sprays is also essential. Impregnated nets, wristbands and ankle bands can be purchased.

Overlanders who frequently live in villages with the indigenous country folk, will probably get the impression that the villagers do not suffer from malaria or other serious diseases and can develop a false sense of security. The problem with malaria in the Asian, African or the South American countries is that practically everyone suffers from malaria in childhood and many children die of it. Anyone who is lucky enough to survive to adult life has developed immunity from the frequent infections. The villagers may give the appearance of being untroubled by the infections and parasitic infestations which are present in their country; in fact their bodies have learnt to live with their problems but in general they suffer from chronic ill health and frequently from chronic malnutrition to such an extent that their life expectancy is far less than it is for the average European, so do not be misguided by initial appearances.

The overlander has not yet developed any of this immunity having lived in a non-malarious area. Hence he or she is like virgin soil to the malaria parasite spread by the night biting anopheline mosquito and he or she has no resistance to infection.

A medical kit

The overlander must take a comprehensive medical bag or a larger one for a party if the organisers are not already providing what is necessary. There is the truly medicinal side of the bag and the sterile equipment content. For a personal bag there should be an adequate supply of disposable syringes and needles, suturing (stitching) packets for severe cuts, transfusion giving sets and small dressings. For a group the bag should contain a larger amount of all the above plus flasks of blood expander (Haemocel and dextro-saline) in case any of the group needs a transfusion and AIDS screened blood is not available. However it is absolutely essential for every overlander to know his or her blood group so that if possible a fellow member in the group could give blood if necessary. Any normally fit, non anaemic, person can give at least one pint of blood. Sterile packing as already mentioned can be obtained from British Airways Immunisation Centres, M.A.S.T.A. at the London School of Hygiene and Tropical Medicine and Trailfinders Medical Advisory and Immunisation Centre at 194 Kensington High Street, London, W.8.

So far as the medicinal contents are concerned, the overlander can be several days' away from adequate medical care so the question of carrying a wide spectrum antibiotic is certainly of great

---

SUMMARY

Advice for overlanders

1 Remember the drug pedlars.

2 Have all possible inoculations well before travel.

3 It is essential to purify water by filtering, *then by* boiling or using sterilising tablets.

4 Insist on essential food hygiene as already described.

5 Maintain full malarial prophylaxis by tablets and general preventive medicine.

6 If you give yourself a course of antibiotics, have a full treatment course of anti-malarials at the same time, as your fever may be due to malaria.

7 Remember to have a medical check-up on return by a suitably experienced doctor.

8 Carry a suitable sterile syringes etc. pack with a covering letter from a doctor.

---

importance with respect to chest infections which are in fact quite common in this type of traveller. An adequate amount of Fansidar or Mefloquine tablets should be included in case of malaria. What must be remembered is that malaria can present an amazing variety of symptoms not only similar to severe influenza but with diarrhoea or even severe chest infection such as pneumonia. If you are a long way from medical advice and antibiotics are thought necessary then a course of antimalarial tablets should be taken along with the antibiotic if you are in a malarial area and in case the fever is due to malaria.

For diarrhoea a capsule such as Imodium is advisable but the most important treatment of severe diarrhoea is replacement of lost fluid, and natural salts (or electrolytes) and sugar. Suitable sachets of salts and sugar in the correct strength can be purchased from chemists. Two such products are Dioralyte and Rehydrat. If the diarrhoea keeps recurring despite 2—3 days of Imodium and sugar/electrolyte treatment medical advice must be sought. Some like to include metronidazole (Flagyl) for the treatment of giardiasis or amoebiasis but without medical advice this can cause problems. Other suggested contents can be found in Appendix C.

A medical check

Finally, it would be an excellent idea if all overlanders had a thorough medical check-up preferably at a tropical medicine centre on return to their homeland. What is absolutely essential is that if they fall sick after the completion of their journey they must tell their doctor where they have been.

11

Don't forget the children

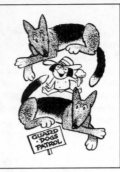

All conscientious parents are concerned about the health of their children and those thoughts come out clearly in young mothers who are about to take their young children overseas, whether on holiday in a warm climate or to live overseas for a longer term.

Immunisation and prophylactics for pregnant women

During the expectant mother's pregnancy, it is considered inadvisable for a woman to be given any "live" vaccines. The live vaccine for yellow fever should not be given to the expectant mother purely for International Health Regulation reasons and a certificate of exemption should be issued. If, however, the mother is visiting a highly endemic area then the risk of yellow fever is greater than the risk of the vaccine, but if possible the vaccination should be delayed until after the first three months of pregnancy. However the need for this precaution is now rare.

The second live vaccine is the oral poliomyelitis vaccine. The original vaccine given by injection is a killed vaccine and so, if a pregnant woman is leaving for a developing country where there is not a satisfactory vaccination programme but where there is poliomyelitis, she should be given a course of the killed injectable vaccine.

Rubella or German measles vaccination is never given during pregnancy when vaccinations against measles and mumps should also not be given.

Cholera and typhoid vaccines are killed vaccines and tetanus is a toxoid so they are not dangerous in pregnancy but, as a general principle, it is best if they are not given in the first three months or at the time of a missed period.

Having covered the immunisations and vaccinations the next most important subject is the prevention of malaria in the pregnant woman. Malaria is regrettably one of the infections which can pass from the mother through the placenta to the foetus. If a mother contracts malaria during pregnancy her baby can be born with malaria. Naturally this is something which must be avoided at all costs, besides the fact that the pregnant woman is likely to have malaria far more seriously than the non-pregnant.

Nowadays, quite correctly, there is a strong movement against pregnant women taking medicaments because of a possible harmful effect on the foetus. However, Paludrine or proguanil and chloroquine are non toxic to the foetus whilst malaria itself is very toxic. If possible, Maloprim should not be taken in pregnancy but if it is, then folic acid must be given as well to prevent maternal anaemia.

Infant health

Breast feeding is even more important for the health of babies in tropical countries than it is for these in developed countries. Many years ago when I was in practice in Nairobi with several colleagues we did a survey of the incidence of gastroenteritis in European children who had been breast fed and bottle fed. The incidence of diarrhoea was appreciably less in the breast fed even up to the age of three years. So every encouragement should be given to a mother to breast feed her babies in the tropics in order to give them a good start in life.

We all know that diarrhoea in infants can be a serious problem, particularly in the developing countries and in warm climates where the general incidence of diarrhoea is far higher and the standards of food hygiene far lower.

As a basic principle all milk and water should be boiled even more thoroughly than in a developed country. If a family has local domestic help then the mother must insist on doing all the food preparation for her babies herself, and she should keep, for them, separate kitchen utensils such as milk saucepans which only she uses and washes herself, and preferably keeps locked away.

One must next consider the vaccinations and inoculations with special respect to children which must be divided into those which may be required by the International Health Regulations and those which are medically recommended.

● **Required by International Health Regulations.** The two concerned are yellow fever and cholera. In general, most countries lay down a minimum age limit of one year for these two vaccinations. However, there are exceptions and when the country lowers the age limit to six or three months or even to no minimum at all then one has to comply with its demands. (Appendix D details these demands by country.)

● **Medically recommended inoculations.** First come those which an infant is given under normal circumstances even when living in a developed country, namely diphtheria, tetanus, poliomyelitis and whooping cough as well as measles, mumps and rubella (German measles) MMR vaccination. As has been mentioned previously it is even more important for all children to have these inoculations when they are going to a developing country because these diseases are still common in such countries. Typhoid vaccination should be given from about the age of two years. As with "overlanders" inoculation against tuberculosis must be seriously considered in all children going to live in developing countries where tuberculosis is still rife. Preferably they should be tested first to see whether they have any immunity against tuberculosis. This is by means of a skin test called a Mantoux test but it is not absolutely essential for this to be done first. In the U.K. this is arranged through the local clinics.

Before one goes any further let us make it quite clear infants and young children do remarkably well in the subtropics and tropics. However, there are obviously certain points of general care that one must stress with regard to small children.

The journey

Let us first start with the journey to the tropics, especially as it is usually by air. Babies are probably the best air travellers of all. When they are small and are on frequent feeds and sleeping a fair amount of the day they are not upset by circadian rhythm problems as with adults. Also their air passages or Eustachian tubes connecting their noses with their ears are comparatively larger and they are less likely to suffer earache. If they do get earache they will automatically cry which clears the air passages so they usefully treat themselves. When they are still young enough to be in a carrycot their transportation is easy because most airlines have fixtures on the "bulkheads" (the partitions dividing up the cabin) to take carrycots. Hence when booking your flight you should inform the airline reservations that you have a baby in a carrycot and they will reserve the row of seats next to the "bulkhead" for you.

Toddlers and older children are a different problem on a flight because they naturally become restless and the conscientious parent becomes concerned lest they are upsetting other passengers. Obviously a certain amount of innocent bribery must be brought into play here and parents should set forth on the journey with a good selection of little presents in the form of suitable toys with which the children can play during the flight, each present being handed out one at a time at suitable intervals to break up the monotony of the journey. Here again most airlines carry a few games on the aircraft but, if there are many children on one flight, there are obviously not enough to go round. The other point is that children frequently want to keep any games with which they are playing and in all fairness the airline cannot be an ever open toy cupboard. Most airlines have their "club" for children which in British Airways is the "Junior Jet Club" and, on joining this, they are given "cut-outs" and other little presents.

It is important to have a light and warm woolly in the hand luggage if you are involved in a night flight because it can become quite chilly in the middle of the night even in the tropics.

On arrival

With regard to acclimatisation it is absolutely essential to maintain fluids in children. This is obviously more difficult to assess than with adults because with their various sizes the amounts vary. However, the principle of watching the colour of the urine is an excellent guide. The addition of plenty of salt in the cooking will also provide some of the extra salt needed.

Clothing is most important with babies and children and the need to avoid nylon and other manmade fibres as described in Chapter Four is essential. With babies, kind relatives in temperate climates will provide little nylon dresses and the like but I regret to say they should not be worn. With young children once they have been in the tropics long enough to have passed the stage of sunburn then it is almost a matter of the less they wear the better, but what they wear must be cotton or principally cotton.

Naturally great care must be taken initially with small children regarding sunburn. For the parts of the body normally covered when one is sunbathing in the Mediterranean or tropical areas a quarter of an hour is plenty on the first day, half an hour on the second, one hour on the third, two hours on the fourth and then increasing by an hour daily. What one must remember is that in these places the sea is warm and children love to play in the sea, in a swimming pool, or in a paddling pool if they cannot swim. Once they are in the water the carefully applied anti-sunburn creams and lotions are washed off and as time is usually forgotten, the trouble starts. A good tip is to wear an old shirt or similar piece of clothing during the first week when in the water. It is incredible how much of the sun's rays in the tropics will filter through so that when it is taken off in the second week there is a suitable basic tan.

With regard to medical problems which may affect children in the tropics, the most common, namely diarrhoea, has already been discussed. Common sense on food hygiene, is obviously the answer and is most essential.

Although we have already discussed the wearing of a minimum of clothing one must mention that children should not run around barefooted because certain worm infections, such as the hookworm, can enter from the earth through the skin of the feet.

The next problem to be considered with special reference to children is malaria. In a malarious area all babies must be given a prophylactic anti-malarial right from the start, especially if they are not being breast fed.

With babies and children there is possibly an indication to move away from the use of the daily proguanil or Paludrine as the best anti-malarial prophylactic for general use. Regrettably proguanil is bitter and hence there is the difficulty of children taking it. However, there are many parents who succeed in getting their children to take proguanil either as it is or with sugar or other sweetening agents such as jam. If they fail then it is essential for them to give the children another prophylactic. The obvious one is chloroquine and there still may be some problems in taking it. There is the disadvantage of it being a weekly tablet and therefore harder to remember but it is obviously up to the parent to see it is not forgotten. However Chloroquine (as Nivaquine) is sold as a syrup (Chapter Eight).

One of the great benefits for children living in warm climates is that they can learn to swim at a young age. However, in countries where there is bilharzia or schistosomiasis they must not be allowed to go off with their friends to swim in the rivers and lakes which are infected. I have mentioned in Chapter Seven which these countries are. Of course with children spending many hours in swimming pools there is the greater possibility of their getting outer ear infections. How to prevent this problem will be mentioned in Chapter Thirteen.

In hot and particularly humid climates the cuts and abrasions which a normally active child collects tend to get infected far more easily than in temperate climates, so they should be suitably cleaned as soon as possible after they are sustained and watched whether they heal satisfactorily.

Despite all the problems I can only reiterate that small children do well in hot climates.

SUMMARY

Don't forget the children — ten times over

1 Breast feed if at all possible.

2 See that the child has all the immunisations possible at the correct age.

3 Anti-malarials are essential from the start in malarious areas.

4 Cook your baby's food yourself.

5 Keep special kitchen utensils for the baby, used and washed only by yourself.

6 Boil all water and milk.

7 Maintain the fluids.

8 Cotton clothes essential.

9 No swimming in rivers, lakes and harbours.

10 Look after minor cuts and abrasions for fear of sepsis.

12

Cold climate comfort

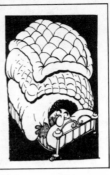

Most people who live in temperate climates decide to go to warmer climates for their holidays. Since developed countries are, in general, in temperate areas businessmen and technical advisers do most of their travelling to warmer climates.

However, there are exceptions to these generalities. There is the increasingly popular winter sports holiday, and businessmen from temperate and warmer areas have to visit the colder countries of northern Europe and northern America. As such we should give a little thought to what helpful advice we can give them. Interestingly, and perhaps surprisingly, some of the principles in keeping warm are the same as those in keeping cool.

We have briefly described the changes which occur in the heart and circulation with heat so we should mention the corresponding changes with cold.

The body's reaction to cold

Basically there is an increase in arterial blood pressure but no change in heart output and little change in heart rate. The increase in blood pressure is due to the narrowing of the small arteries, or arterioles, so significantly reducing the blood flow to the skin and superficial muscles and hence maintaining warmth. The heart muscle works harder and needs an increase in oxygen. Because of this the person who suffers from pain over the heart (angina) feels far worse in the cold. Similarly in those with arteriosclerosis, or hardening of the arteries, the blood flow to the hands and feet is impeded and excessive chilling of these occurs.

Insulation and your clothes

When describing clothes to keep one cool, I stressed the point of wearing string vests under the shirt or top garment in order to establish a layer of air to encourage perspiration. Similarly a layer of air next the skin in cold weather provides a layer of insulation which keeps the body warm. For the person who travels from warm climates to cold climates or vice versa by far the best undergarments to wear are cotton string vests and pants because they keep you cool in the heat and warm in the cold.

Following on the principle of keeping a layer of air around one as insulation one must mention the point that clothes must be loose and have plenty of room. At no time should they be tight, in particular shoes, because when they are, the air insulation is lost and coldness ensues.

The principle of a layer of insulation is seen in the wearing of wet suits for diving, particularly in the Antarctic, where the temperature of the water is approximately 0°C or 32°F: water gets into the suit and a layer of still water acts as an insulation. A further example of the importance of insulation can be seen in the actual variation of clothing for wear in cold climates although in principle they are similar. With the Eskimo the clothing is composed of skins and consists of two layers, the main insulating layer being a smock and trousers made of fur with only a light layer worn underneath. When the Eskimo enters his igloo he removes his furs and wears little due to the warmth of the igloo, but the light layer underneath aids the air insulation. Clothing worn by modern explorers and soldiers also consists of numerous layers of fairly ordinary clothing. String vests, woollen vests and several pullovers with an outer layer of near windproof material is the principle of their cold weather wear.

Clothes, as already mentioned, must be loose-fitting and it is far better for them to be a size too large rather than small. Tight fitting clothes prevent there being the insulating layer of air. This is most important with gloves and shoes, and it is far better to wear fingerless mittens rather than fingered gloves as they give far more movement to the fingers and far better insulation. Cold fingers occur in tight gloves, not in good sized mitts, and again it is a sound principle to wear a lightweight glove or preferably a mitten inside the heavier weight outer mitten. The inner glove can be cotton, silk or lightweight wool. In R.A.F. night bombers during the war, there was no basic heating and the temperature was frequently below zero. Crews were provided with three pairs of gloves, an innermost silk glove, a middle lightweight wool glove and an outer heavy mitten. Radio operators and navigators frequently had to take off their outer heavy mittens to operate their instruments but the silk and lightweight wool were able to give them satisfactory insulation whilst they were conducting their duties.

Similarly, it is most important that there is plenty of room in shoes or boots. Tight fitting footwear will cause cold toes which may lead to frostbite. Skiers and mountain climbers find it best to wear an inner pair of cotton or lightweight woollen socks and over them a heavier, preferably oiled, wool sock giving the insulation. Naturally the boots must be at least half a size and probably a whole size bigger than you would normally wear.

A final point on clothing is that it should fit closely, but not too tightly at the extremities, so that cold air cannot get in and chill the body. Hence gloves should fit over the sleeves and socks or boots should fit over the trousers. A snug fit at the neck helps to contain body heat within the upper garment.

In most cold climates bed linen is usually in the form of a duvet or continental quilt, now becoming popular in Britain. Their light weight and insulation properties are far better for keeping one warm at night than heavy blankets tucked in under the mattress.

Keeping dry

A most important point in keeping warm in cold climates is keeping clothes dry. Once clothes become wet the water in them can freeze and the insulating powers are lost. This principle is of importance both against the wet coming from the outside in the form of rain and also from inside the clothing in the form of perspiration. It is most important not to get too overheated by excess clothing and perspire excessively because subsequent cooling can freeze the perspiration with dire results, which is another reason for not wearing manmade fibres next to the skin. If there is a possibility of getting wet, it is most important to wear a waterproof layer on the outside. In addition, even if the clothes have become wet, an outer waterproof layer will prevent the enormous heat loss that can occur with evaporation.

Headgear

Ears should be covered as they can become frostbitten easily and as such, suitable headgear affording protection to the ears is essential.

It is a wise thing to keep the head covered in the cold but it is even more necessary to keep the ears covered.

Hypothermia

What is the basic first aid answer to this most unpleasant complaint and to generalised chilling? In the past one has, on the one hand, been told not to warm people up too quickly and on other occasions that rapid warming is the answer. We now think that each method has its proper place. The point here is that the treatment for acute hypothermia or chilling is different from chronic hypothermia (which so sadly occurs in the elderly who cannot afford adequate heating). Most experts now consider that anyone who has been exposed acutely to cold should be warmed up as rapidly as possible and rapid immersion in hot water is the immediate answer. In fact, mountain rescue teams immerse those whom they rescue in a hot bath, clothes and all. With elderly people who have grown cold over a period of time the answer is to warm them slowly.

SUMMARY

Cold climate comfort

1 Wear loose clothes with plenty of room.
2 Keep clothes dry.
3 Layers of clothes with air in between add to insulation.
4 Acute frostbite — warm rapidly.
5 Chronic hypothermia — warm slowly.
6 Sun and snow — sunglasses essential.
7 If winter sporting, remember health insurance is essential.

Further points for skiers

Many people experience cold climates when they visit the mountains for winter sports, in particular skiing. One of the pleasures of skiing is that of enjoying it whilst the sun shines. This however has its snares and delusions because, although it will appear to be still very cold, the sun is extremely strong and the problems are far greater because of the maximum reflection of the sun's rays from the white snow.

The subject of types of sunglasses is considered in the next chapter. For anyone who is winter sporting where there is strong sun and snow the wearing of sunglasses is virtually essential and must be seriously considered. The problem of sunburn, which is common in winter sports, is also discussed in the next chapter.

A further point regarding the skiing holidaymaker which is most important and fully discussed in Appendix A is the essential need to take out an adequate insurance policy to cover accidents and also airfares home which might involve returning as a stretcher case.

Altitude acclimatisation and acute mountain sickness

Wherever you are if you climb high enough you will reach a cold climate. Mount Kilimanjaro 200 miles from the equator has permanent snow on its summit at just under 20,000 feet. The subject of altitude acclimatisation and acute mountain sickness is discussed in Chapter Four.

13

Other problems, summary and final advice

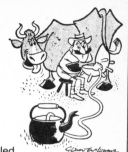

All milk should be boiled

We have now covered most of the medical problems which may trouble the modern traveller, but there are just a few points I would like to stress which do not really come in to any category which we have discussed.

Sunglasses

The views concerning sunglasses are many and various. Certain criticisms of them by an eye specialist a few years ago reached the daily press with the result that many people began to wonder whether they were harmful. In fact, by the time his very sensible remarks reached the press, they were distorted: the point he tried to make was that it was bad to wear sunglasses if the light was dull as it put a strain on the eyes. We have all seen the pop or film stars who wear dark glasses in this manner to prevent them getting wrinkles around the eyes. This is, of course, wrong.

However, in conditions of glare it is completely different, and sunglasses are of inestimable value. One must further remember that reflection of the sun is strong with snow, and also on the white sand of tropical beaches where the sea is very clear or where there is a coral reef with pools. Hence the wearing of sunglasses in these types of surroundings is beneficial and good quality sunglasses, made by proven firms, should be purchased. With good quality lenses there is an even transmission throughout the visual spectrum so that there is no loss of colour appreciation, which in fact can well be increased by removing the glare. Naturally there is a very wide range of tints and, with this, depth of tints. Different people like different colours.

For the person who has to wear glasses all the time it is frequently advisable to get his or her own prescription made up in tinted lenses. Unless there is a medical reason for the lenses to be tinted, they cannot be obtained under the N.H.S. As these glasses are for use in hot climates lightweight frames should be used and plastic lenses are light and efficient. The only thing to remember is that plastic lenses scratch far more easily and that sunburn lotions and creams, insect repellents and some cosmetic creams can make the lenses opaque if they get smeared on them.

The table lists good quality lenses and with their name I have added the colour and the approximate percentage of light transmitted through the lens.

Polarised lenses are of particular benefit in giving protection against reflected glare from a horizontal surface. They are thus normally good for fishermen and vehicle drivers provided there are no distractions from patterns in toughened windscreens. Equally they are not so good for situations in which the glare comes at one from many angles such as in mountainous snow-covered surroundings.

Name	Colour	Light transmission
Crookes Alpha	Hardly perceptible	82%
Crookes A2	Pale blue	79%
Crookes B	Greenish smoky	51%
Crookes B2	Deep greenish smoky	26%
Softlite 1	Pale flesh	87%
Softlite 2	Slight flesh	80%
Softlite 35	Flesh	47%
Rayban 3	Deep green	32%
Cruxite 1	Pale flesh	85%
Solbar 1	Very pale flesh	87%
Solbar 2	Pale pinky	80%
Solbar 3	Light pink	73%

Of the tinted plastic lenses popular varieties are:

Neutint 1½	Medium smoke	55%
Rose	Rose	85%

In the last few years a new type of tinted lens has been produced, namely the photochromic lenses. These lenses change colour according to the amount of light falling on them and are therefore for sunshine use, as the protection varies according to the need. They can be made up to anyone's particular prescription as well but they are not available, as yet, in plastic lenses. The principle is that embedded in the glass are a large number of crystals which change colour when exposed to sunlight in a similar way to photographic film. With brown lenses they are silver halide crystals. Once you move out of the bright lights the crystals turn back to their original form and the glasses become lighter again. However, they are not permitted for driving in Italy.

Here again there are different makes of these lenses but the following are reliable.

Umbramatic (Zeiss)	Darkens to a dark sherry
Reactolite (Chance Pilkington)	Darkens to brown, blue or grey
Photogray	Darkens to grey

As well as these there are vacuum-coated tinted lenses which have the advantage of an even depth of tint over the entire lens whatever the prescription. These types are sold under the names of Astor, Grisolux and Rosalux.

Coral

Many of the finest tropical beaches which are fast becoming so popular for holidays with their guaranteed sunshine have coral reefs usually just offshore. This applies to the beautiful beaches south of Mombasa. Because the reef is just offshore the breakers are dispersed before reaching the beach, leaving excellent safe bathing for children.

Where these coral reefs are present there are usually pools in the reef abounding with highly-coloured tropical fish, which naturally attract the bathers. However, great care must be taken with coral because it is sharp and abrasive, causing unpleasant cuts and abrasions. Frequently bits of the coral break off in powdery form, getting embedded in the abrasions, causing slow healing with some discharge from the area. Anyone who walks on a coral reef must wear light shoes such as gym shoes.

A pure thin rubber shoe may tear on the coral and can be unsatisfactory. For those who are snorkelling in the pools, great care must be maintained not to swim into too shallow water, thus rubbing the knees or elbows on the coral and causing abrasions. One must also remember that time passes rapidly whilst snorkelling and, if the back is exposed above the surface, severe sunburn can ensue.

Ear irritations

Another problem with coral is getting the fine granules in the outer ear, where they cause intense irritation which usually makes the sufferer rub it or scratch it. The result is that the individual develops a discharge from the outer ear which, like the abrasions, is slow to heal.

With regard to an irritating or discharging outer ear, known as external otitis, there must be a warning about unhygienic swimming pools. There are many scattered around the world, some even at the best hotels, that are not nearly as hygienic as they should be. The water is not changed frequently enough, and the purification system is unsatisfactory, and as a result, external otitis can develop. In the airline medical world we have found that the incidence of this trying condition can be minimised with the use of antiseptic ear drops before and after swimming, wiping out the drops on both occasions. Mercuric chloride — one in a thousand parts in spirit — ear drops can be used.

Skin conditions

Two skin conditions must be mentioned.

The first are the fungus infections, of which by far the most common and the one which will be discussed goes under the long name of *epidermophytosis,* but known to most as Athlete's Foot, Foot Rot, Hong Kong Foot, or Mango Toe. Common all over the world it is known in most residential schools and communal bathing establishments in the U.K. An important factor in the cause and frequency of athlete's foot is in the last sentence, communal bathing establishments. The fungus revels in moisture and therefore it flourishes in the tropics where there is excessive sweating of the feet due to the heat. This is naturally made far worse if the potential sufferer wears non-absorbent nylon socks. However, a lot can be done to prevent the spread of athlete's foot.

1   The feet must be dried thoroughly with a rough towel every time they become wet, such as after a bath or in particular after getting out of a swimming pool.

2   If it does appear, it is good to use one towel for the feet and another towel for the rest of the body to prevent spread.

3   The wearing of cotton socks is best and nylon should never be used. If infection does occur and cotton socks are worn, they can be boiled after use, so killing the fungus which breeds in the little

flakes of skin which come off from between the toes.

4   The use of an anti-fungul or fungicidal dusting powder, which should be dusted into the socks, can be obtained from any chemist without prescription. This powder should be used whenever anyone travels to warm climates, whether they have athlete's foot or not.

5   In the event of developing athlete's foot a fungicidal ointment or paint should be used. I personally think a paint is best because it has a surer action and is less messy. There is one, Monphytol, on sale in the U.K. which I find particularly successful.

The final skin condition which must be mentioned is common in South Africa and Florida and occurs in the rest of Africa, the Caribbean, and in the East: *Larva Migrans,* a creeping eruption or creeping itch. It is caused by the larva of one of several types of worms burrowing into the skin, usually of the foot, leaving an irritating raised line as it progresses, usually at the rate of ½″ to 1″ per 24 hours. It can be treated quite simply, either by a doctor freezing the end of the line by local anaesthetic, or by the giving of thiabendazole. More important is that it can be prevented by wearing shoes so that the larvae do not burrow into the feet, or lying on a towel rather than directly on the sand.

Summary: forty-one points for your safety and comfort

I have reviewed the majority of the medical and semi-medical problems which may assault the modern traveller. I have tried to show that all those mentioned can be prevented by a little basic knowledge and common sense.

To finish, I will summarise the various points in the previous chapters. They are all precautions which are easy to take, and cause the absolute minimum of discomfort or annoyance. By taking them, I think that overseas business trips or your holiday in the sun can be made so much more safe and enjoyable.

All these 41 points are most important but naturally some of the points concern certain areas of the world, and some concern others. As I have said repeatedly, they are all simple, they are all common sense, and between them they can provide the basis of a pleasant trip.

Most of them however, can be included in ten basic commandments which I will give as a final summary. Please do not think that these ten commandments cover eveything everywhere. The 41 points are obviously more comprehensive.

1   See that all your inoculations are up to date well before the date of your flight.
2   Plan your flight well in advance; if possible a day flight and/or arrive at your usual bedtime.
3   Not too hectic a last 24 hours before flight.
4   Try to cut smoking before and in-flight.
5   Moderate your alcohol in flight.
6   Moderate your food in flight.
7   Maintain your fluids in flight — not sparkling drinks.
8   Wear loose-fitting and comfortable clothes and shoes.
9   Keep light but warm clothing at hand.
10 A 24-hour rest period on arrival after a 5-hour time change. Never go straight into a meeting or reception.
11 Carry a mild aperient and a quick-acting sedative with you and keep all regular medicaments, including insulin and the necessary syringes and needles, in your hand luggage.
12 Avoid fatigue during acclimatisation.
13 Maintain your fluids: 1 pint per 10°F per 24 hours or 2 litres + 1 litre for every 10°C = 4 litres at 20°C and 5 litres at 30°C.
14 Maintain your salt with your fluids.
15 Never wear nylon.
16 Go easy with the sun at first on the principle ¼ hour, ½ hour, 1 hour, 2 hours, etc., per day.
17 Use good quality sun creams and lotions. The higher the Sun Protection Factor number the greater the protection.
18 Take two pills of Sylvasun (not in pregnancy) daily for the first two weeks if available (or one Roavit capsule).
19 The truly sun-sensitive must use a barrier cream.
20 Boil all drinking water and milk.
21 Be very careful of shellfish and preferably see them alive first.
22 All cooked food to be well-cooked and recently cooked.
23 All fruit including tomatoes peeled.
24 Lettuces and unpeeled fruit sterilised by chloramination — no water-cress.
25 No left-overs or food on display.
26 Beware of local ice creams — only eat those from large firms.
27 Drink mineral waters from reputable bottlers.
28 Avoid fly-infested restaurants.
29 Never eat underdone or uncooked meat or fish.
30 Never walk about in bare feet, other than on the sea shore.
31 Never bathe in rivers or lakes unless you *know* they are schistosomiasis free, or in harbours.

32   Keep yourself well-covered after dark.
33   See you have good mosquito-proofing either on the window or over the bed.
34   Use an insect-repellent on your skin frequently.
35   Use an insecticidal spray in your bedroom.
36   Take your recommended anti-malarial from one week before you set forth until 28 days after you leave the malarious area.
37   If you are bitten by an excited dog wash the bite thoroughly and go at once to a doctor or hospital.
38   If you keep a dog in the tropics, de-flea, de-tick, and de-worm it regularly.
39   In a snake area always take a torch out at night and tuck your trousers tight round your ankles.
40   Always shake a shoe before putting it on.
41   With a snake bite, reassure the patient, clean the wound, and go to hospital. Do not incise.

SUMMARY

Ten commandments for overseas travellers

1 After a flight with a 5-hour time change, rest for 24 hours.

2 See your foods are well cooked.

3 Peel all fruit and be careful with salads and ices.

4 Do not buy any food or drink from street hawkers.

5 Go easy with the sun at first and use good quality creams or lotions.

6 Maintain your fluids and salt.

7 Take anti-malarials from one week before reaching a malarial area until four weeks after leaving.

8 Boil drinking water and milk.

9 Never wear nylon in the heat.

10 No bathing in unknown rivers and lakes or harbours.

If you become ill on your return or within a month of your return from an overseas trip tell your doctor where you have been.

Appendix A
Overseas medical costs and insurance

Although every care has been taken over the following information no responsibility can be accepted for any errors or inaccuracies.

It is when the British subject is taken ill on holiday or business abroad and that person is not covered by a sickness policy that he or she realises what a wonderful institution the much maligned National Health Service really is.

After over 40 years of the N.H.S. the general public takes it all for granted and, regrettably, often travel abroad oblivious of the financial risks to which they are laying themselves open.

Although the majority of us are critical in one way or another of the N.H.S., free treatment, with the exception of small statutory charges, is available to all. Illnesses or accidents incurred by visitors to the U.K. are also covered by the scheme, though no-one from abroad may bring their illnesses in with them and have them treated under the scheme.

Before the time when the U.K. joined the European Economic Community or Common Market it was always strongly advised that every traveller from the U.K. should take out adequate sickness insurance cover. When we joined the E.E.C. the majority of us thought that this would no longer be necessary on visiting E.E.C. countries when we think of the way we offer the N.H.S. to our visitors, even before we joined the E.E.C. However, there are so many complications and variations between the member countries as to what one has to do to get any entitlement that it is still far better to take out insurance cover. Besides, there are definite deficiencies in the entitlement.

The cost of bringing a person back to the U.K. in the event of illness is **never** covered by the special arrangements with other E.E.C. countries or with the non-E.E.C. with whom we have these special arrangements. If you are staying near the border of an

E.E.C. country or another with whom we have arrangements you might be transferred to a hospital over the border into a country in which we have no arrangements for treatment. This can happen when skiing in northern Italy and transfer to a hospital in Switzerland might be advisable. Further if you are driving in any of the countries listed and you have an accident, you may not be covered for medical treatment. Make sure you check with your insurance company and/or motoring organisation before you leave the U.K.

Let us consider first the problem of those who are visiting the E.E.C. countries, then look at countries which, although outside the E.E.C., have agreements with the U.K., and finally we shall discuss insurance policies.

Travellers to E.E.C. countries

Up to and including June 1982 those self-employed and not employed were not entitled to any financial cover in the E.E.C. countries. This was relevent to wives and children as well. However, this was changed from 1st July 1982, when they became entitled, correcting a grossly unfair situation, and certainly not before time.

You must anticipate being ill by filling in forms before you travel and taking a card with you when you go abroad.

You must go to your local office of the Department of Health and Social Security, any Employment Exchange or Post Office *not more* than six months before you travel and get a form CM1. This form is attached to an SA30 obtainable from a D.S.S. office. Form CM1 has six questions all of which have to be answered and when completed returned to the nearest Social Security Office. If your answer to Question 6 (which concerns whether you are going abroad once or repeatedly) is "no" you will then be issued with a form E111 certifying that you and your dependants are entitled to benefits under the E.E.C. regulations. If your answer to Question 6 is "yes" you send the form to D.S.S. Overseas Branch, Newcastle-upon-Tyne, NE98 7YX. If your dependants are travelling alone and you are entitled, they are automatically entitled; but you must complete a CM1 to obtain an E111 for them in advance of their travel. However if you visit the E.E.C. countries frequently, on business for instance, you must get another form which is valid for a longer period, again from Newcastle. The only E.E.C. countries where you do not require an E111 are Denmark, Eire, Gibraltar and Portugal. In the other countries if you do not have an E111 you will not get the financial benefits.

Note that any financial reimbursement to which you are entitled must be obtained within the E.E.C. country where you are sick *before you leave* because it is almost certain you will not be able to obtain it later. This applies particularly in Denmark and Germany. Throughout the E.E.C. countries there is generally no provision for refund after leaving the country concerned. At best, there is likely to be a long delay before any settlement. If you cannot get a refund whilst abroad write explaining why to D.S.S., Overseas Branch, Newcastle-upon-Tyne, NE98 1YX; or if you live in Northern Ireland, to D.S.S. Medicines and Food Control Branch, Annex A, Dundonald House, Belfast BT4 3TL. Enclose your E111 and the originals of medical bills, receipts and other medical documents. If treatment was given in France, before sending for repayment you must at the end complete and sign the *feuille de soins,* and attach to it the *vignettes,* which are the small identification stamps supplied with medicines. If you were prescribed medicines in Italy the price tags must be sent with your claim. If treatment was given in Belgium send the *Attestation de soins donnés.*

How to get treatment
Remember your E111 is essential in all E.E.C. countries except Denmark, Eire, Gibraltar and Portugal. In fact, it is of great value to have extra photocopies of the E111 because in France, Germany and Holland the doctors will require these for their records. Procedures for getting treatment are now described, country by country.

Belgium

Administrative authorities: Addresses of local offices may be obtained from the head offices.

Auxiliary Fund for Sickness and Invalidity Insurance (La Caisse Auxiliare d'Assurance Maladie-Invalidité), 10 Boulevard Saint-Lazare, 1030 Brussels. Tel. 182300.

National Alliance of Christian Friendly Societies (Alliance Nationale des Mutualités Chrétiennes), 131 Rue de la Loi, 1040 Brussels. Tel. 358080.

National League of Federated Liberal Friendly Societies of Belgium (Ligue Nationale des Federations Mutualistes Libérales de Belgique), 19—25 Rue de Livourne, 1050 Brussels. Tel. 384154.

> Since re-writing this appendix the method of obtaining the E111 has been simplified.
>
> Visit your Post Office and get the form 'Health Care for visitors to E.C. Countries. This contains an application form for your E111. Answer all the necessary questions and when you have completed it take it to the Counter Officer at the Post Office who will stamp it and so authorise it. It is of no value unless stamped by the Post Office.
>
> N.B. E111 basically only covers emergency treatment.

National Union of Federated Non-Party Friendly Societies of Belgium (Union Nationale des Fédérations Mutualistes Neutres de Belgique), 145 Chaussée de Charleroi, 1060 Brussels. Tel. 388300.

National Union of Federated Professional Friendly Societies of Belgium (Union Nationale des Fédérations des Mutualités Professionelles de Belgique), 13 Rue Boduognat, 1040 Brussels. Tel. 332188.

National Union of Socialist Friendly Societies (Union Nationale des Mutualités Socialistes), 32 Rue Saint-Jean, 1000 Brussels. Tel. 136470.

The addresses of the local offices of the above organisations should be available in the local telephone directory.

If treatment from general practitioner is required

1 Go straight to doctor and show the E111.
2 Pay the doctor but obtain a receipt.
3 Take prescription to a chemist, obtain a receipt and keep a copy of prescription. In some areas doctors may provide medicine but you should still obtain a receipt.
4 Take receipts with E111 to local office of one of the organisations mentioned above. The refund will probably be in the neighbourhood of 75 per cent.
5 Receipts should be stamped on the official form — *Attestation de soins donnés.*

If hospital treatment is required

1 Go to the local office of one of the organisations with E111 and staff will advise where treatment can be received and authorise part payment.
2 If you have to go to hospital in an emergency show them the E111 and ask the staff to arrange authorisation of part payment

through local offices.
N.B. If you are obtaining treatment in Belgium for an established industrial injury received in the U.K., tell the authorities this.

Denmark

Administrative authority: Social and health divisions of the local councils. (Kommunens Social — OG Sundheds-forvaltning). Addresses of local offices may be obtained from local post offices or from the Administration of Social Security, Holmens Kanal 7, Copenhagen.

If treatment from a general practitioner is required
1 Take your passport along to the doctor of your choice, as an E111 is not required in Denmark. Names of doctors registered with the Danish Public Health Service may be found in the telephone directory or from the social and health division of the local council. If the doctor charges a fee, obtain a receipt and apply for repayment at the local council.
   In general, the cost of specialist treatment arranged by a general practitioner will also be paid by the local council.
2 Take your prescription to a local chemist. If the chemist is on the scheduled list, on production of your passport a reduced charge will be made which is not refundable.

If hospital treatment is required
Free treatment is normally arranged through the general practitioner.

Accident and sudden illness
Ambulances can be summoned by dialling 000 in an absolute emergency. In general, contact should first be made with a general practitioner. Strict rota systems are worked by G.P.s and the practitioners' emergency service number can be found in the telephone directory under *Laegevagten*. Urgent general treatment can be obtained on part payment, on production of passport.

France

Administrative authority: Local Sickness Insurance offices (La Caisse Primaire d'Assurance-Maladie). Office in most towns.

Address may be obtained from the Town Hall (Hotel de Ville). In Paris: Caisse Primaire Centrale d'Assurance-Maladie de la Region Parisienne, Centre 461. 84, Rue Charles Michels 93525, St Denis. Tel. 820.61.05. Dept. Services des Relations Internationales.

If treatment from general practitioner is required

1 First take E111 to local Social Security office, who will issue a sickness document *(feuille de maladie)*.

2 Take this form to a doctor or dentist, pay for the service but see the payment is entered on the form. Similarly, at the chemist the cost of medicine must be entered on the form and a copy of the prescription given. The medicine containers have detachable stamps (name and cost of medicine). Detach and stick these to the *feuille*.

3 In the event of not being able to carry out (1), take the E111 to a doctor who should provide the sickness document.

4 Finally take E111, sickness document and copy of the prescription to the Social Security office. Repayment is usually 75 per cent of fee and 70 per cent of prescription.

If hospital treatment is required

1 Outpatient treatment must be paid for and reclaimed later.

2 If the doctor advises hospital treatment he will give you a certificate of emergency *(attestation medicale d'urgence)*.

3 This certificate is shown at the hospital and enquiries should be made as to public and approved private hospitals.

4 The sickness insurance office will pay 80 per cent of the costs direct to the hospital.

In some approved private hospitals you may be required to pay the medical fees in advance. If the hospital is not "bound by convention", you may have to pay the cost of accommodation. If this is so, apply to the sickness insurance office with your E111 before leaving the district for refund of their share of the costs, but these will not always be refunded in full.

5 If you go direct to a hospital without seeing a doctor first you must ask the hospital to get a certificate from the sickness insurance office authorising their acceptance of costs.

Germany

Administrative authority: Local sickness insurance offices (Allegemeine Ortskrankenkassen A.O.K.). Open Monday to Friday. Mornings only. Addresses from town hall and post offices.

If treatment from general practitioner is required

1 First take the E111 to the local sickness insurance office *(Krankenkassen)* which will provide a sickness document *(Krankenschein)* and a list of doctors and dentists who practise within the scheme.

2 Then take the document to the doctor of your choice who will treat you without charge.

3 The chemist will charge a small fixed amount, not recoverable, for each item.

4 If you visit a doctor without a sickness document show the E111. He will charge you but if you obtain a sickness document subsequently and take it to him within ten days, he will repay your fee.

N.B. Not all doctors and dentists are in the insurance scheme; hence it is best to obtain the list first. *Alle Kassen* on the doctor's or dentist's name plate signifies he practises within the insurance scheme.

If hospital treatment is required

1 Obtain a certificate from a G.P. *(Notvendigkeitsbescheinigung)* and take it and the E111 to a local sickness insurance office. They will issue a further certificate *(Kostenubernahmeschein)* to enable you to obtain free hospital treatment (third class). This is then taken to the hospital.

2 If attendance at hospital is a matter of urgency take the E111 to the hospital and ask the staff to obtain the further certificate.

N.B. It must be remembered the free entitlement is only for third class grading. For an established industrial injury follow-up treatment, carry on as above but inform the local sickness insurance office that it is an industrial injury. If you go into a convalescent home you will be charged for accommodation.

Gibraltar

Enquire at your hotel, the Health Centre, Casemotes or the Medical and Health Department, St Bernard's Hospital.

1 Treatment under the local medical scheme is available at the Health Centre on payment of a nominal fee.

2 Your U.K. passport must be produced stamped with a temporary resident's permit or with a cruise ship's embarkation card.

3 Non-British subjects must produce an E111.

4 A small charge is made for each item of medicine.
5 Full charges for dental treatment except in normal working hours Monday — Friday; extractions can be obtained at St Bernard's Hospital for a nominal fee.

Greece

Administrative authority: Social Insurance Foundation I.K.A., 8 Aghia Constantinan Street, Athens; or local offices *(Upokotastinata)* or branches *(Parioutimalta)*.
1 Procedures are the same as for Greek nationals.
2 Long waits should be expected both in the local I.K.A. offices and in surgeries or hospitals. Hospital wards are crowded, with poor nursing services and, in general, you have to provide your own food and laundry services. If, in view of this, you elect for private treatment, then you will have to pay for everything and medical insurance is essential.

If treatment from a general practitioner is required
1 Go to the I.K.A. office and show your E111. They will direct you to an insurance doctor or dentist and you will not be charged.
2 Take a prescription to any chemist showing your E111, where you will be charged 20 per cent.

If hospital treatment is required
The I.K.A. office will arrange free treatment, after you have been seen by the doctor. If you go direct to the hospital show your E111 and inform them you are entitled to free treatment under the I.K.A. scheme.
N.B. If you are in a remote part of Greece or on a small island there will be no I.K.A. office. You will have to pay for private treatment. *Before leaving* Greece you must apply to the *nearest* I.K.A. office personally or by post for a refund, producing your E111, all receipted bills and any other documents. The refund will be not more than 50 per cent. *Private insurance cover in Greece is therefore essential.*

Irish Republic

Administrative authority: Eight local health boards.
Medical care is provided free of direct charge. An E111 is *not*

necessary but make it clear you wish to be treated under the E.E.C. Social Security Regulations. On receiving a medical service you will have to complete a form giving nationality and place of residence, also stating that you are employed in the U.K.

If treatment from a general practitioner is required

1   On consulting a doctor it is essential you ask for treatment under the E.E.C. regulations. If you do not request this he has every right to charge a fee which is not refundable. The list of doctors participating in the scheme can be obtained from the offices of the local health boards or from the telephone directory under "Health Boards". Under these regulations there is no fee to pay as the doctor is paid by the Health Board.

2   Provided that the prescription is on the official form there will be no charge from the chemist either.

If hospital treatment is required

This would normally be arranged through the general practitioner. There are no charges in public wards at hospitals participating in the scheme. There are direct charges for semi-private and private rooms when consultants charge as well, as in the U.K.

Italy

From January 1st 1980 a National Health Service *(Servizio Sanitario Nazionale)* was instituted. However integration can be slow. Where the N.H.S. is established the authority is the local health unit *(Unita Sanitaria Locale)*. If this is not established then the authority is the S.A.U.B. *(Struttura Amministrativa Unificata di Base)*. Information can be obtained from either of these sources. (The S.A.U.B. was previously known as the I.N.A.M.)

If treatment from a general practitioner is required

1   Take your E111 to the local office.

2   You will be given a certificate of entitlement but ask to see a list of the scheme's doctors and/or dentists.

3   Take the certificate to the doctor or dentist and you will be treated free of charge.

4   If you need prescribed medicines take the prescription to the chemist but you will have to pay a standard charge.

N.B. If you do not first get the certificate of entitlement you will have to pay the doctor and may have difficulty getting the money back, and even if you get a refund it will only be partial. If you are charged in full for the medicines keep the price tags since without these you will not get a refund.

If hospital treatment is required

1   If the doctor thinks you need hospital treatment he will give you a certificate *(Proposta di ricovero).* This entitles you to free treatment at certain hospitals, a list of which is kept in the local office.

2   If you cannot contact the office show your E111 to the hospital authorities and ask them to get in touch with the local office regarding your right to free treatment.

Luxembourg

Administrative authority: National Sickness Insurance Office, 10 Rue de Strasbourg, Luxembourg. Local agencies at Battenbourg, Clervaux Dierkirch, Differdange, Dudelange, Echternach, Esch/Alzette, Grevenmacher, Larochette, Mersch, Petange, Redange-sur-Attert, Remich, Rumelange, Steinfort and Wiltz.

If treatment from general practitioner is required

1   First take form E111 to local sickness office, which will provide you with a sickness document.

2   Take the form to a doctor who will make a charge for which you must obtain a receipt.

3   Take the prescription to the local chemist, who will again charge you, so obtain a receipt.

4   Take your receipts to the local sickness office. You will be fully refunded for the doctor's fee but may have to pay a small percentage of the chemist's charges.

If hospital treatment is required

1   First obtain a certificate from a doctor, which you should take to the local sickness office with your E111. Hospitalisation is normally free. In an emergency you can go direct to a hospital and ask staff to contact the local sickness office.

N.B. For an established industrial injury follow-up treatment you must contact the Insurance Association for Accidents (L'Association d'Assurance contre les Accidents), 1 Rue Zithe, Luxembourg. Tel. 20511.

Netherlands

Administrative authority: Netherlands General Sickness Insurance Fund (Algemeen Nederlands Onderling Ziekenhuis — A.N.O.Z.), 56 Kromme Nieuwe Gracht, Utrecht. Tel. 0/0-317541.

If treatment from a general practitioner is required
1   Take your form E111 to a doctor or dentist but you should ask whether he or she is affiliated to the A.N.O.Z. fund. Hand over a photocopy of your E111. Medical treatment is free and there is part payment for dental treatment.
2   If drugs are not provided by the doctor, take the prescription to an approved chemist where again there will be no charge, if you give the chemist a photocopy of your E111.

If hospital treatment is required
1   It is advisable first to obtain the authority for free treatment from A.N.O.Z. in Utrecht. This is best done through the doctor.
2   In an emergency, treatment can be obtained without prior authority of A.N.O.Z., but this must be cleared within two days and again a photocopy of your E111 is needed.
N.B. For treatment for an established industrial injury the procedure is as above.

Portugal (including Azores and Madeira)

Administrative authority: In Portugal information can be obtained from the Regional Health Service Offices (Administracao Regional de Saude); in the Azores the Regional Social Security Directorate in Angra do Heroisimo; in Madeira Regional Social Security Directorate in Funchal.

An E111 is not necessary for a U.K. citizen as a U.K. passport is sufficient. If not a U.K. citizen a medical care booklet in exchange for the E111 must be obtained from the relative administration office (see above).

If treatment is required from a general practitioner
Show your passport to the doctor (or medical care booklet) and ask to be treated under the E.E.C. arrangements, but you must make sure the doctor works from the state scheme health centres (Centro de Saude). A charge may be made and in Madeira if you consult

a private doctor you will have to pay. Ask for the official (green receipt) and claim a refund from the nearest appointed bank, but only a very small refund will be made.

Prescribed medicines — you will probably have to pay 20—65 per cent of cost and for some you will have to pay the full amount. Dental treatment is limited under the state scheme and you will have to pay for it without refund.

If hospital treatment is required

Show your passport (or E111) to the hospital authorities and ask to be treated under E.E.C. arrangements. You may have to pay for secondary examination e.g. X-rays and laboratory tests.

Spain (including Balearics and Canary Islands)

Administrative authority: Information can be obtained from a provincial office (Director Provincial) or local office (Agencia) of the National Social Security Institute (Instituto Nacional de la Sequidad Social) I.N.S.S.

If treatment from general practitioner is required

Immediately after arrival in Spain you take your E111 to an office of the I.N.S.S. and exchange it for a book of vouchers. You have to see a doctor practising under the Spanish health care system and the names of such doctors are given in the voucher book. You may have to travel some distance to find such a doctor either in his surgery (Consultario) or the health centre (Ambulatario). Hand a voucher to the doctor. You must seek treatment within the stated hours and he or she will then treat you free of charge.

Take the prescription to any chemist (Farmacia) where you will have to pay 40 per cent of the cost although medicines are free for E.E.C. pensioners.

If hospital treatment is required

The doctor will arrange hospital treatment if necessary. If you go direct show your voucher and ask to be treated as an I.N.S.S. Patient. You have to go to a state hospital and be in a public ward to get free treatment.

N.B. In most holiday resorts only a limited service is available under the Spanish scheme. Private medical insurance is strongly advised.

Summary of arrangements for E.E.C. countries

There are obvious problems in relying on E.E.C. medical arrangements which are inferior to what the N.H.S. offers the visitor. To summarise:

1 First, before setting out, a form CM1 must be obtained, completed and returned to a D.H.S.S. office or Post office.

2 This will provide you with an E111 which must be taken with you.

3 Children over 16 not in full-time education and all children of 19 and over must obtain their own E111.

4 E111s are, however, not necessary in Denmark, Ireland, Gibraltar and Portugal.

5 In France, Germany and Italy the patient or one of his family has to visit the local social security office first to obtain a permit before seeing a doctor.

6 In Belgium, France, Luxembourg, and sometimes in Denmark, the doctor's fee must be paid and a receipt obtained. Money must be reclaimed from the local authority before leaving the country.

7 In Belgium the patient is repaid approximately 75 per cent; in France 75 per cent of the general practitioner's fees and 80 per cent of the hospital's.

8 In Germany, Holland, Italy and Spain G.P. treatment is free, but only from certain panel doctors.

9 Free hospital treatment is only available in certain hospitals. In Germany this is officially described as 'third class', in Ireland as "public" and in Portugal and Spain as state or official.

10 In Greece it is strongly advised to take out medical insurance.

11 Spain and Portugal have recently joined the E.E.C. but the benefits are limited and insurance cover is essential.

Travellers to non E.E.C. countries

Outside the E.E.C. the government has agreements for financial assistance in certain countries for urgent medical attention. Briefly the details are as follows:

Anguilla

It is necessary to provide proof of residence in the U.K. such as N.H.S. medical card or driving licence. Basically only minor emergency treatment is free. All hospital in-patient and out-patient treatment plus dental treatment are charged. Ordinary general practitioner treatment is obtained at outpatient clinics. Ambulances are also charged for.

Australia
Proof of U.K. residence is essential and a U.K. passport or N.H.S. card plus a temporary entry permit must be produced.

The basis of free treatment is the Medicare scheme in which you have to register. It is best to register at a Medicare office on arrival but you can do it after you have received treatment.

Hospital treatment is free. You pay for prescribed medicines and ambulance services but some general practitioners give treatment under the Medicare scheme, but you must claim any repayment before leaving Australia.

Austria
In-patient treatment in public wards of public hospitals is usually free but you may have to pay ten per cent of the total cost for dependants. All other medical services have to be paid for. It is necessary to show your U.K. passport. You may have a right to Social Security benefits.

British Virgin Islands
The only people who are entitled to any free treatment are those over 70 and school age children. Proof of U.K. residence and age (N.H.S. card or U.K. driving licence) is essential. All other visitors are charged at rates similar to residents.

Bulgaria
Hospital and other medical and dental treatment is free if you are normally living in the U.K. and show your U.K. passport and N.H.S. medical card. A charge is made for prescribed medicine.

Channel Islands
Alderney and Guernsey: hospital, general medical care and emergency dentistry are free but there is a small charge for some prescribed drugs. Ambulances are free in Guernsey. There is no out-patient department at Guernsey General Hospital. Proof of residence in the U.K. may be required, such as driving licence or N.H.S. medical card.

Jersey: hospital treatment and ambulances are free. A family doctor type clinic is held at the General Hospital on Monday—Saturday mornings inclusive, May to September; and Monday, Wednesday and Friday, October to April. This clinic is free and there is also a casualty outpatient department. A charge is made for prescribed drugs, for dentistry and for attendance at a doctor's surgery.

Sark: medical treatment is free. There is no hospital and transfer is to Guernsey in an emergency.

Czechoslovakia

Hospital and all medical care is free but prescribed medicines are subject to some charge. You must show your U.K. passport.

Falkland Islands

Proof of U.K. residence, such as N.H.S. medical card or U.K. driving licence is necessary, when basically everything is free, including all medical treatment, both hospital and G.P., dental, prescribed medicines and ambulances.

Finland

U.K. passport is necessary. Consultation at a Health Centre is now free. Some other charges may be refunded but claims must be made before leaving Finland.

Hong Kong

U.K. passport and N.H.S. card must be produced. Emergency treatment at certain hospitals and clinics is free. A list of these establishments is available from Department of Health I.R. (H) Alexander Fleming House, London, SE1 6EY. Small charges are made for other services and treatment. What must be remembered is that calls by hotel doctors are always chargeable and frequently added to your hotel bill.

Hungary

Treatment in doctor's surgeries, polyclinics (large health centres) and hospitals is free. There is a flat rate charge for prescribed medicine but dental and ophthalmic treatment has to be paid for. U.K. passport required.

Iceland

U.K. passport necessary. If not a U.K. national but resident in the U.K. N.H.S. medical card is sufficient. Hospital in-patient treatment and emergency dental treatment for children between the age of 6 and 15 are free. Hospital out-patient treatment, G.P. attendance, prescribed medicine, other dental treatment and ambulance services are charged for.

Isle of Man
Basically as in the U.K. You pay charges for dental treatment and prescribed medicines. Contraceptive pills are not free.

Malta
If your stay is less than 30 days then treatment for an emergency at a Government hospital is free. Treatment in a doctor's surgery or a non-Government hospital has to be paid for. A U.K. passport or tourist permit is required for free treatment.

Monserrat
Proof of U.K. residence in form of N.H.S. medical card or U.K. driving licence.

Only persons over 65 and children under 16 years of age are entitled to free treatment and that is only at Government Institutions. School-age children are entitled to free dental treatment. Family-doctor type treatment is available at Government clinics and in the hospital in-patient and out-patient treatment and hospital accommodation has to be paid for as well as prescribed medicines, dental treatment and ambulance travel.

New Zealand
In-patient treatment in public hospital and, in general, prescribed medicines along with dental treatment for children under 16 are free. Payment has to be made for out-patient treatment at hospitals and attendance at a doctor's surgery along with certain drugs. However, cash benefits can be obtained from the New Zealand Department of Health to reduce the charges. It is essential to ask the doctor and/or the hospital whether these benefits have been deducted from the bill. If not, a claim must be made at the local health office. Your U.K. passport is essential.

Norway
Hospital in-patient treatment is free as also is travel by ambulance. You have to pay for out-patient and other medical treatment including general practitioner attention so it is essential to obtain a receipt for payment. You take the receipt and your U.K. passport to the local Norwegian Social Insurance Office (*Tryg de kasse*) and they will give you a refund of about 80 per cent of your total outlay. *However you must reclaim this money before you leave Norway.* You have to pay for prescribed medicines but some dental treatment is free.

Poland

Hospital and other medical treatment is free if you normally live in the U.K. but it is necessary to show your N.H.S. medical card. There is a charge for a visit by a general practitioner. With prescribed medicines there is a 30 per cent of cost charge if it is obtained from a public pharmacy. Some dental treatment is free.

Romania

Hospital and other medical treatment is free but you have to pay for prescribed medicine supplied by a public pharmacy. Some dental treatment is free. You have to show your U.K. passport and evidence that you normally live in the U.K., such as your N.H.S. medical card or your driving licence.

St Helena

Proof of U.K. residence either in form of U.K. passport or N.H.S. medical card. Hospital out-patient treatment in normal clinic times is free. This includes normal family doctor type attention. Hospital in-patient treatment, prescribed medicines, dental treatment and ambulance travel are all charged for.

Sweden

Hospital in-patient treatment, including prescribed medicines in hospital, and ambulance travel, are all free. A reduced charge is made for out-patient treatment, all other medical treatment and prescribed medicines obtained from outside pharmacies. A 50 per cent fee is charged for dental care. It is necessary to show your U.K. passport.

Turks and Caicos Islands

Proof of U.K. residence in the form of a N.H.S. medical card or U.K. driving licence is necessary. All treatment to those under 16 or over 65 is free. On Grand Turk Island dental treatment at the dental clinic, prescribed medicines and ambulance travel are also free. On the outer islands medical treatment at government clinics and prescribed medicines are free but there are no hospital services on the outer islands. Hospital in-patient treatment and other treatment at the Town Clinic are charged for on Grand Turk Island.

U.S.S.R.

Hospital and other medical attention is free but there is a small charge for prescribed medicines. Some dental treatment is free. It is necessary to show your U.K. passport.

Yugoslavia

In-patient and out-patient hospital treatment is free as is attendance at health centres if available, but prescribed medicines warrant payment. Some dental treatment is free. It is essential to show your U.K. passport. However, if taken ill on holiday you may have a right to sickness benefit.

It must be remembered that calls made to a hotel by the "Hotel Doctor" are chargeable.

Insurance policies

It can be seen from the foregoing sections that every country differs in the medical treatment it offers to visitors and that they all fall short of what the U.K. offers visitors. Remember that the above regulations in general only apply to U.K. citizens normally resident in the U.K. and not to other members of the Commonwealth and other countries.

The author feels strongly that with all the above-mentioned complications and variations, it is a far sounder plan with only one exception, to take out an insurance policy. Regrettably, the elderly pensioner and his wife who are covered by the E.E.C. arrangements may not be able to obtain any insurance cover. Certain insurance companies enforce a maximum age but in general if you pay more you can get cover. Some demand double premium from 65 years, some double from 70 years and some treble from 75 years. They may also ask for a fitness certificate from your doctor. Some companies only demand the excess for age for worldwide and not for European cover only. In general, there is a clause of having to pay the first £25 but, if on visiting an E.E.C. country and using your E111, they cancel the clause.

There is a further point in favour of the insurance policy. Accident or sickness may cause delay in returning home. Many policies allow for this, and cover incidental expenses and cancellations due to delays so incurred.

If it is decided to take out a medical expenses insurance policy, the first point to remember, as with all insurance, is that the sum insured must be adequate. Most inclusive tours now include a medical expenses insurance. The cover provided in these "included" policies used to be quite inadequate but recently they have improved greatly and in general are now satisfactory.

The medical cover is at least £250,000 but many policies give cover for £500,000 or £1,000,000. This may seem a tremendous amount of money but hospitalisation in the U.S.A. can cost well over £1,000 per day and an air ambulance back from the U.S.A. could cost over £25,000.

People travelling other than in an inclusive tour must take out individual policies produced by various companies. There are specific points to remember.

1   Most policies exclude the first £25 of the expenses: however a few only exclude this £25 for children and elderly: some do not lay down the excess if you use the E111 and E.E.C. facilities in these countries.

2   Most policies cover accidents in general but not winter sports accidents unless the appropriate premium has been paid which is usually double, but may be even three times as much. This addition must be requested.

3   Some policies do not cover mini-trekking or safaris unless an additional payment is added to the premium.

4   The problems for the over 65s have already been mentioned and must be seriously considered by elderly couples who visit such countries as Spain in the winter when the hotels are cheap, sometimes on a fairly long term to avoid heating costs in the U.K. It is absolutely essential for them to take out adequate insurance cover.

5   Some policies do not include delays or disruption benefits unless an extra premium is paid.

6   Nearly all policies divide areas of the world into:
   a) U.K., Northern Ireland and the Isle of Man.
   b) Europe including countries of North Africa bordering the Mediterranean, the Azores, Canary Islands, Madeira and the Channel Islands.
   c) worldwide.

Naturally the premiums increase through 1 to 3.

7   British United Provident Association, Private Patients Plan, Western Provident Association and similar organisations provide cover for hospital cost overseas, but it must be remembered that as overseas costs are so much higher that the cover might not be complete. In addition these organisations do not cover G.P. attendance, emergency dental treatment or cancellation and associated costs which are necessary.

Types of policy

There are basically two types of policy available:

1   The optional Travel Insurance Policy is one in which the

traveller sets the amount of cover he wants for baggage, medical cover, personal accident, or personal liability himself. It is really only practical for people who need special arrangements as it is far more expensive. General Accident are probably the firm to approach if you want this type of policy.

2   The usual policy which is most suitable is the inclusive policy which should include baggage and personal money, personal accident, cancellation and curtailment charges, medical and emergency expenses, personal liability, delayed departure, and legal expenses and advice. Some give an extra financial benefit if hijacked. The author, with his insurance consultant, looked at nearly a dozen policies and going on the principle of a minimum cover for baggage and money of £1,500 and for medical expenses of £500,000 we found the Cornhill Insurance seemed to offer the best cover with the General Accident very close to it. These are of course personal views. For 17 days Cornhill were charging £33.60 and General Accident for 18 days £33.70 on a worldwide basis. The benefits were fairly similar. Naturally European cover only is cheaper.

In addition to the above policies, holders of American Express and Diners Club credit cards can arrange insurance cover through these organisations. American Express do it through Medex, which has listed doctors around the world whom it recommends and whose bill it guarantees to pay. The advantage of this scheme is that you do not have to pay a bill and then reclaim from the insurance as it is paid automatically. Medex will give cover for winter sports for an additional premium. Diner's Club have a similar policy through Europe Assistance. Both organisations give these policies free if you have charged your travel tickets through these organisations. For the regular air traveller the International Airline Passengers Association Incorporated have a full insurance policy covering all the usual sections.

So it can be seen that there are many variations in insurance and many opportunities to be insured.

The two constant factors are that sickness insurance is absolutely essential when travelling abroad and it must be adequate. People who have travelled to the U.S.A. without insurance cover have been known to have to sell their house to pay for medical expenses.

The frequent business traveller has to consider a different policy and must take out one which gives cover for a whole year. Annual policies normally cover holidays within the year and discounts are granted when including the wife and children. Annual policies however usually lay down a maximum period for any one trip which is sometimes 60 and generally not more than 91 days. If you decide on taking out a policy for a 'one-off basis' rather than an annual policy is must be realised that it only covers one trip. In other words if you take a policy for 21 days, return after ten days, and then have to return to the U.S. After four days for three days you are not covered for your second trip, although within the 21 days. N.B. The small print must be read.

One has to be careful of some insurance policies provided by the plastic card companies if you buy your air tickets through them. Some only cover compensation for accidents which is not the same as cover for medical expenses if you fall ill abroad. Some 'business' policies cover the cost of replacement of an employee if he or she falls sick overseas. What I have stressed in all cases previously is that the amount of financial coverage for overseas sickness, particularly in the U.S.A. must be adequate.

Organisations which specialise in annual policies for business travel are Norwich Union, Commercial Union, Europe Assistance, Bishopsgate, Extrasure and Marcus Hearn.

Remember whatever policy you take read the small print.

Medical facilities for U.K. Nationals in E.E.C. countries

	Belgium	Denmark	France	Germany
Administrative authority	La Caisse Auxilaire d'Assurance Maladie-Invalidié	Local authorities	La Caisse Primaire de Sécurité Sociale	Allgemeine Ortskrankenkassen
Is E111 necessary?	Yes	No	Yes	Yes
Is certificate from admin. auth. necessary to see doctor?	No	No	Yes	Yes
Is doctor free?	Pay and obtain receipt	Sometimes pay but obtain receipt	Pay and obtain receipt	Yes
Is cost repaid by admin. auth.?	75%	Full repayment	75% G.P. 80% Hospital	n/a
Is chemist free?	Pay and obtain receipt	Reduced charge	Pay and obtain receipt	Small fixed charge
Is cost repaid by admin. auth.?	75%	Not repaid	70–90%	Not repaid
Is certificate from admin. auth. necessary before going to hospital?	Yes	Arranged through G.P.	Inform admin. offices	(1) cert. from doctor, then (2) cert. from admin. offices
Is hospital free?	Pay and obtain receipt	Yes	Pay and obtain receipt	Yes
Is cost repaid by admin. auth.?	Approx. 75%	n/a	80%	n/a N.B. Third class accommodation

Medical facilities for U.K. Nationals in E.E.C. countries

	Gibraltar	Greece	Ireland	Italy
Administrative authority	Health Service	I.K.A.	Local Health Boards	Unita Sanitario Locale and S.A.U.B.
Is E111 necessary?	No but UK passport is necessary. Non-British subjects require E111	Yes	No	Yes
Is certificate from admin. auth. necessary to see doctor?	No	Yes	No	Yes
Is doctor free?	Nominal fee	Yes	Yes	Yes
Is cost repaid by admin. auth.?	No	n/a	n/a	n/a
Is chemist free?	Nominal fee	20% charge on showing E111	No charge if approved	Free or small charge
Is cost repaid by admin. auth.?	No	No	Not repaid	Not repaid
Is certificate from admin. auth. necessary before going to hospital?	No	Yes	Arranged through G.P.	S.A.U.B. and list of approved hospitals
Is hospital free?	Free in public wards. St Bernard's Hospital	Free in public wards but provide own food	Yes, in public wards of certain hospitals	Yes
Is cost repaid by admin. auth.?	n/a	n/a NB Take out insurance	n/a	n/a but only certain hospitals

Medical facilities for U.K. Nationals in E.E.C. countries

	Luxembourg	Netherlands	Portugal (inc. Azores and Madeira)	Spain (inc. Balearics and Canaries)
Administrative authority	National Sickness Insurance Offices	A.N.O.Z.	Information obtained from Offices of Administracao Regional de Saude in Portugal. Similar offices in Angra do Heroisimo in Azores and in Funchal in Madeira	Instituto Nacional de la Seguridad Social (I.N.S.S.)
Is E111 necessary	Yes	Yes	UK Passport. Other E.E.C. subjects require E111	Yes
Is certificate from admin. auth. necessary to see doctor?	No	No	Other nationals need to exchange E111 for medical care book	Exchange E111 for book of vouchers on arrival from above offices
Is doctor free?	Pay and obtain receipt	Yes	A charge may be made. In Madeira you pay but obtain official receipt. Repayment at bank	Yes: if you have book of vouchers and obtain treatment from state scheme Dr (names in book)
Is cost repaid by admin. auth.?	Full refund	n/a	In Madeira repayment at bank with official receipt	No
Is chemist free?	Pay and obtain receipt	No charge	Usually charged 20–65%. May be 100%.	Charged 40% Pensioners free
Is cost repaid by admin. auth.?	Partly repaid	n/a	No	No
Is certificate from admin. auth. necessary before going to hospital?	(1) cert. from doctor, then (2) cert. from Admin. Offices	Obtain Authority through G.P.	No — but ask to be treated under E.C. arrangements	Book of vouchers
Is hospital free	Yes	Yes	You may have to pay for X-rays and laboratory work	Yes in State Hospital in public ward
Is cost repaid by admin. auth.?	n/a	n/a	No. Hospital or Dr must be told you wish to be treated under E.C. arrangements	No. If you do not obtain vouchers it is very rare for any cost to be repaid.

Medical treatment for visitors to non E.E.C. countries

Country:	Free:	Charges	You must show	Other details
Anguilla	Minor Emergency Treatment	All hospital treatment and accommodation. Dental treatment Medicines Ambulances	NHS medical card or UK Driving Licence	Family doctor type treatment available at outpatient clinics but a charge is made
Australia	Hospital Treatment	Treatment at some doctors surgeries. Prescribed medicines. Ambulances	UK Passport or NHS medical card plus temporary entry permit	Need to enrol at local Medicare Office. Some charges may be refunded by Medicare. Claim before you leave
Austria	In-patient treatment in public wards of public hospitals	10% of in-patient treatment of dependants. All other medical services, including treatment at hospital out-patients dept and doctor's surgery	UK passport	See the paragraph about entitlement on page 135
British Virgin Islands	Hospital and other medical treatment for school children and those over 70 years	Other visitors charged for everything as residents rates	NHS medical card or UK driving licence	
Bulgaria	Hospital, medical and dental treatment	Prescribed medicine	UK passport, NHS medical card	

Medical treatment for visitors to non E.E.C. countries

Country:	Free:	Charges for	You must show	Other details
Channel Islands	If you stay for 3 months or less:			
Alderney and Guernsey	Hospital and other medical care. Emergency dental treatment. Ambulance travel (Guernsey)	Some prescribed	Proof of residence in the UK may be required (e.g. your driving licence)	No out-patient department at the Guernsey General Hospital (Princess Elizabeth hospital)
Jersey	Hospital in-patient + out-patient treatment. Ambulance travel	Prescribed medicine. Treatment at a doctor's surgery. Dental care		
Sark	Medical treatment			No hospital. Emergency cases taken to Guernsey.
Cyprus				
Czechoslovakia	Hospital and other medical care	Prescribed medicine	UK passport	
Falkland Islands	Hospital and other medical treatment. Dental treatment. prescribed medicine. Ambulance		NHS medical card or UK driving licence	

Medical treatment for visitors to non E.E.C. countries

Country:	Free:	Charges for	You must show	Other details
Finland	Consultation at health centre	Hospital treatment. Prescribed medicine. Dental treatment (for adults). Ambulance travel	UK passport	For some private care charges may be partially refunded by Sickness Insurance Institution. Claim at local office before leaving
Hong Kong	Emergency treatment at certain hospitals and clinics*	Small charges are levied for all other services and treatment	UK passport and NHS medical card	*List available from D.H.I.R. (H) A. Alexander Fleming House SE1 6BY. If hospital or clinic is not on list full charge will be made
Hungary	Treatment in hospitals, polyclinics and at a doctor's surgery	Prescribed medicine (flat rate charge) dental & ophthalmic treatment	UK passport	
Iceland	Hospital in-patient. Emergency dental treatment aged 6—15 years	Hospital outpatient. Other medical treatment. Other dental treatment. Medicine. Ambulance	UK passport or NHS medical card if not UK national	
Isle of Man	Treatment as in UK National Health Service	Prescribed medicine (flat rate charge per item). Dental treatment		

Medical treatment for visitors to non E.E.C. countries

Country:	Free:	Charges for	You must show	Other details
Malta	If your stay is for less than 30 days: treatment in an emergency at Government hospital	Treatment at a doctor's surgery and in non-Government hospitals	UK passport or tourist permit	
Montserrat	Treatment at Government Institutions for under 16 years and over 65 years. Dental treatment for school age children	Hospital in-patient and outpatient. Hospital accommodation. Most prescribed medicines. Dental treatment. Ambulance	NHS medical card or UK driving licence	Family doctor type treatment available at Government clinics and hospital casualty dept. Charge is made
New Zealand	In-patient treatment in public hospitals. Prescribed medicine (Usually). Dental treatment for children under 16	Other treatment at hospitals and at a doctor's surgery. Certain drugs. Cash benefits from New Zealand Department of Health reduce charge to patient	UK passport	Ask hospital or doctor whether benefit has been deducted from the fee claimed. If not, claim the benefit at the local health office
Norway	Hospital in-patient treatment. Ambulance travel. Some dental treatment. Drugs for specific chronic conditions	Doctor's visit (e.g. hotel doctor. 30% cost of prescribed medicine by a *public* pharmacy)	UK Passport	Ask for a receipt and take it with UK passport to local Norwegian Social Insurance Office (Trydekasse). You must claim before you leave Norway

Medical treatment for visitors to non E.E.C. countries

Country:	Free:	Charges for	You must show	Other details
Poland	Hospital and other medical treatment. Some dental treatment	Doctor's visit (e.g. hotel doctor). 30% cost of prescribed medicine supplied by a *public* pharmacy	NHS medical card	
Romania	Hospital and other medical treatment. Some dental treatment	Medicine supplied by a public pharmacy	UK passport and NHS medical card or driving licence	
St Helena	Hospital treatment in outpatient clinics in normal clinic times	Hospital in-patient treatment. Dental treatment. Ambulance. Prescribed medicines	UK passport or NHS medical card	Family doctor type treatment is available at the hospital out-patient clinic
Sweden	Hospital in-patient treatment. Prescribed medicines in hospital. Dental treatment for children.	Outpatient and other medical treatment, and prescribed medicine from a pharmacy. Part of cost of ambulance travel.	UK passport	Travelling expenses to hospital may be partially refunded. Claim from local Health Office in Sweden

Medical treatment for visitors to non E.E.C. countries

Country:	Free:	Charges for	You must show	Other details
Turks and Caicos Islands	All treatment for those under 16 years or over 65 years **On Grand Turk Island** Dental treatment at dental clinic. Ambulance. Prescribed medicines **On Outer Islands** Medical treatment at Government clinic. Prescribed medicines	Hospital in-patient treatment. Other medical treatment at town clinic	NHS medical card or UK driving licence	No hospital service available on the outer islands
USSR	Hospital and other medical treatment. Some dental treatment	Prescribed medicine	UK passport	
Yugoslavia	Hospital and other medical treatment. Some dental treatment	Prescribed medicine	UK passport	See the paragraph about Entitlement on page 139

Appendix **B**
Purification of water

Water for drinking can be purified by three methods: boiling, filtration and chemical disinfection.

Boiling

However impure the water adequate boiling is by far the most effective and safest method of purifying it even if there are "foreign bodies" present and it looks filthy and discoloured. Boiling destroys all forms of disease organisms whether they are bacteria, spores, cysts or ova. Follow this method:

1 The water should be brought to the boil and maintained mildly bubbling for five minutes. It should then be transferred to adequately cleansed and sterilized containers.

2 The best ones are ordinary clean glass bottles such as empty gin and squash bottles. They should be immersed in a saucepan of water and brought to the boil for five minutes, and then allowed to cool.

3 The recently boiled water for drinking should then be transferred to the newly sterilized bottles, and the mouth of the bottle covered. The principle is that when you boil water it drives out the contained gases so giving it a flat taste. Even if the container is closed some absorption of gases takes place in the partially filled bottle and flavour is regained.

4 If a refrigerator is available place the partly filled container in it.

5 With refrigerators, one must remember that, when ice cubes are made, boiled water must be used. If not, when the ice cubes dissolve in the drink, the purified water is automatically made impure.

Filtration

The main purpose of water filters is to remove all suspended matter from the water. This makes drinking water far more palatable but does not necessarily purify it completely. There are several kinds and makes of filters.

The usual process is that of the water seeping through "filter candles" which have very fine pores (e.g. Chamberland L2, Selas 015, Berkefeld, Mandlers, Metafilter and Stella filters). They remove all suspended matter and frequently organisms which cause disease if they are living in the suspended matter.

No mechanical method of purification of water is proof. What must be remembered is that the filters must be frequently inspected to see that they have no cracks or leaks through which unfiltered water could pass. They must also be kept clean and not allowed to become coated with solid matter. They should be scrubbed under running water once a week such that all solid matter is removed, and should then be boiled for 20 minutes.

There are other filters containing silver (Sterasyl, Katadyn, and Metafilter) which, as well as filtering the water, carry out some sterilization of the water. These filter candles do not require boiling and as they are portable with a handpump they can be of great value to travellers such as overlanders.

However, plain filtration is never as fool-proof as adequate boiling, and to be 100% safe one must follow filtration by boiling. This is especially important if the filtration has been left to staff. Regrettably many people seem to think that you should boil the water and then "filter" it. This is absolutely wrong, because if the "filters" are dirty, the water loses its purity. It is quite simple: if you *boil* before you filter, you B before F and you are a B.F.

Great advances have been made in the efficiency of water filters over the last few years. Where in the past they were excellent at removing foreign bodies, sediment, and the like, they were far less satisfactory in removing bacteria. With technical improvements some new filters are reported to be effective in removing bacteria and other infective organisms.

Katadyn Products Inc. of Wallisellen, Switzerland produce the Katadyn Pocket Filter, useful for the hiker or the camper and particularly the overlander. It is 24 cms (10") in length and 6 cms (2½") in width (about the size of a two cell torch). It has attached to it a 50 cm (20") suction hose fitted with an intake strainer to eliminate coarse debris. It also has a cleaning brush and it packs into a zippered soft carrying case. No chemicals are used and, unlike chemical methods, it works equally well with turbid water which it clarifies. It can produce ¾ litre (one and a quarter pints) per minute of safe drinking water. Its cost is in the neighbourhood of £140 but it is an extremely sound product. It can be obtained from Norman,

37 Townsend, Welsford, Grantham G32 3NX.

A small filter is produced by Pre Mac (Kent) Ltd., 103 Goods Station Road, Tunbridge Wells, Kent TN1 2DP. It works on the principle of iodine salts rather than chlorine or silver and the filtered water is tasteless. It is small and cheap and costs around £8. Its main limitations are that it only filters and sterilizes half a cupfull at a time but the result is immediate. The second point is it can only be used for a certain number of filtrations. The makers state filters 500 litres which is about 2000 cupfuls. It has been tested in a leading laboratory in England and the bacterial result was excellent. M.A.S.T.A. at The London School of Hygiene and Tropical Medicine provide a more sophisticated model at around £30.

Chemical disinfection

There are several methods but the basis of most is the Halogen group, namely chlorine and iodine. We are used to the taste of chlorine in water, whether it is in the crude and excessive form of chlorine in swimming baths or in the normal water supply, especially in times of drought when there is chlorination for safety reasons. Two forms of tablets to chlorinate and purify water are Halozone and Sterotabs (Boots). The directions are on the packets but the basis is to over-chlorinate and then to add other tablets to "detaste" the excess chlorine.

Katadyn, the Swiss firm which make the Pocket Filter, also produce a sterilizing tablet based on silver, like their filter. It is chlorine free and does not affect the taste of the water. It can be used for the disinfection of containers and utensils. It is reputed to preserve water for one to six months if the water is kept in a properly sealed and stored container. It can be purchased in powder form as well as tablets and is called Micropur.

Water sterilising powder (stabilised bleach) or Chloramine T tablets can be used for fairly large quantities of water.

In the U.S.A. Potable Aqua tablets are available. These are an iodine based tablet. The advantage is that iodine is effective in killing amoebic cysts as well as bacteria. If these tablets are not available then 2% tincture of iodine can be used, adding ten drops to one litre of water which is left to stand for half an hour. What must be remembered is that neither chlorine nor iodine is effective if the water is cloudy when it must first be filtered.

Appendix C
Suggested 'medical bag'
for travellers

Those marked with an asterisk must be obtained with a doctor's prescription.

Prophylactic anti-malarial tablets	Proguanil (Paludrine) Chloroquin (Nivaquine, Avlochlor, Resochen, Aralen) *Maloprim Mefloquine (Lariam)
Sedative	*Temazepam *Diazepam
Aperient	Senokot or Dorbanex
Pain or fever reliever	Soluble Aspirin or Paracetamol
Indigestion tablets	Gelusil or Polycrol Asilone
†Salt tablets	Slow sodium or effervescent salt tablets
Motion sickness tablets	Dramamine, Phenergan Stugeron
Throat lozenges	Bradosol or Strepsils
Diarrhoea Treatment	*Imodium capsules. Electrolyte and fluid replacement salts in sachets:- Dioralyte, Rehydrat

†It is better to take added salt on food than salt tablets.

Antiseptic ointment	Cetavlex cream
	Fucidin cream
Ointment for stings	Caladryl
Water purification tablets	Halozone, Sterotabs or
	Chloramine T or Tincture of
	Iodine
Insect repellent	Skeet-O-Stik, Autan
	Jungle Formula

Various first aid dressings

Insecticidal aerosol spray

Good Quality Sunglasses

Good quality sunburn lotion or cream not oil, with adequate S.P.F. number

Anti-AIDS kit containing sterile syringes and needles, suture material, transfusion giving sets etc. with doctor's covering letter.

For the backpacking overlander who is away from medical treatment for several days it may be necessary to include an antibiotic such as tetracycline. If the traveller runs a fever in a malarial area and takes a course of the antibiotic he/she must take a course of antimalarial treatment such as Fansidar in case the fever is due to malaria.

N.X.T. International of 17 Clarence Street, Belfast BT2 8DY Northern Ireland produce The Dentowise Travellers Kit which costs approximately £8 including post and packing. The compact Dentowise kit allows the user to easily replace a dislodged crown, or cap or bridge and to also provide a temporary cavity filling or dressing. The kit has a shelf life of five years if unopened. One kit per person is essential to prevent cross-infection. It is highly recommended. The kit is approved by the British Dental Association but it must be stressed that the emergency repairs carried out by using the kits are of a temporary nature only and that professional help must be sought as soon as possible afterwards.

Appendix D
Legally required vaccinations and immunisations for countries, and their climates

In general, the following requirements do not apply to transit passengers who are not leaving the airport. An asterisk (*) against the word "transiting" refers to passengers who leave the airport.

It must be remembered that these legal requirements are for cholera and yellow fever immunisations only. The medical need for typhoid, tetanus and poliomyelitis immunisations and gamma globulin for hepatitis is not mentioned in this section. That is fully discussed in Chapter Two on immunisation.

Please note that infected areas and endemic areas are not necessarily the same. Yellow fever infected areas are as below. Yellow fever endemic areas are as indicated on the maps on pages 15 and 16. When there is a minimum age limit it is stated.

Cholera infected areas
(at time of going to press)

In Africa
Algeria, Angola, Benin, Burundi, Cameroon, Côte d'Ivoire, Ghana, Guinea (Rep.), Kenya, Liberia, Malawi, Mali, Mauritania, Mozambique, Niger, Nigeria, Sao Tome and Principe, Tanzania, Zaire, Zambia.

In Asia
India, Indonesia, Malaysia, Nepal, Vietnam.

In S. America
Ecuador, Peru

Yellow fever infected areas
(at time of going to press)

In Africa
Angola, Cameroon, Gambia, Ghana, Guinea (Rep.), Mali, Nigeria, Sudan, Zaire.

In S. America
Bolivia, Brazil, Colombia, Ecuador, Peru.

Requirements and climate — by country

Paragraph A states the current vaccination requirements, and paragraph B gives a resume of the country's climate.

Vaccination requirements for various countries are liable to change at short notice and whilst every care has been taken with the following information, it is given only as a guide for travellers, and the author and publishers cannot accept responsibility. Final confirmation can be obtained by contacting the respective Embassies or High Commissions.

Afghanistan
A. Yellow Fever — if arriving within 6 days after leaving or transiting* infected areas.
Recommended malaria prophylaxis below 2,000m in May through November. Chloroquine resistance reported.
B. Hot in the summer (July-August). Cold in winter. Rainy season March—April.

Albania
A. Cholera — if arriving within 5 days after leaving or transiting* infected areas (children under 6 months exempt).
Yellow fever — if arriving within 6 days after leaving or transiting* infected areas (children under one year exempt).
B. Mediterranean type. Fairly dry on coast but cooler and wetter inland.

Algeria
A. Yellow fever — if arriving within 6 days after leaving or transiting* infected areas (children under one year exempt).
Malaria prophylaxis recommended March through November in Saharan regions.
B. Mediterranean on coast with hot summers and mild winters. Hot and dry inland. Rainfall October — May.

Andorra
A. No vaccinations required.
B. Mediterranean in the summer but snow and sunshine in mountains in winter.

Angola
A. Yellow fever — if arriving within 6 days after leaving a transiting* country with infected areas (children under one year exempt).
Malaria prophylaxis is essential throughout the country throughout the year. Chloroquine and sulphadoxine/pyrimethamine resistance reported.
B. Tropical. Hot and humid. Little rain at coast; torrential in mountains. Luanda very hot with cool evenings.

Antigua and Barbuda
A. Yellow fever — if arriving within 6 days after leaving or transiting* infected areas (children under one year exempt).
B. Subtropical summer but some wind. Rain August—November.

Argentina
A. Nil demanded from anywhere.
Malaria prophylaxis: in rural areas below 1200m, October through May.
B. Subtropical in north. Subantarctic in south. All variations in between. Buenos Aires can be very hot and humid in summer (December and March). Rain evenly spread throughout the year.

Australia
A. Yellow fever (persons without valid vaccination certificate — if required — may be subject to quarantine) if arriving within 6 days after leaving or transiting infected areas (children under one year exempt). Passengers suffering from a quarantinable disease may be also subject to isolation in a quarantine station.
B. Practically every variation of climate to a cool temperate climate in Melbourne and Hobart. Humid temperate in Brisbane and Sydney and Mediterranean in Perth and Adelaide.

Austria
A. Nil demanded from any country.
B. Temperate — cold at altitude in the winter. Rain heaviest April and November.

Bahamas
A. Yellow fever — if arriving within 7 days after leaving or transiting* infected areas (children under one year exempt).
B. Subtropical. Fairly high humidity. Rainfall May, June, September, October.

Bahrain
A. Yellow fever — if arriving within 6 days after leaving or transiting* infected areas (children under one year exempt).
B. Summer July—October. Very hot and humid. Rest of year mild to warm, but may be cold in January and February. Rainfall November to April but slight.

Bangladesh
A. Yellow fever — if arriving within 6 days after leaving or transiting* infected areas or any part of one of the following countries:
Africa: Angola, Benin, Botswana, Burkina Faso, Burundi, Cameroon, Central African Republic, Chad, Congo, Côte d'Ivoire, Equatorial Guinea, Ethiopia, Gabon, Gambia, Ghana, Guinea, Guinea-Bissau, Kenya, Liberia, Malawi, Mali, Mauritania, Niger, Nigeria, Rwanda, São Tomé and Principe, Senegal, Sierra Leone, Somalia, Sudan (south of 15°N), Tanzania, Togo, Uganda, Zaire, Zambia.
America: Belize, Bolivia, Brazil, Colombia, Costa Rica, Ecuador, French Guiana, Guatemala, Guyana, Honduras, Nicaragua, Panama, Peru, Surinam, Trinidad & Tobago, Venezuela.
Malaria prophylaxis is essential throughout the country throughout the year. Chloroquine resistance reported.
B. Hot with high humidity. Monsoon June—September. Best months January and February.

Barbados
A. Yellow fever — if arriving within 6 days after leaving or transiting* infected areas and countries situated in endemic areas (children under one year exempt).
B. Semi-tropical. Maximum temperature varies little — 80°F. Rain June—November. Heaviest in August and November.

Belgium
A. Nil demanded from any country.
B. Temperate.

Belize
A. Yellow fever — if arriving within 6 days after leaving or transiting* infected areas.
Malaria prophylaxis is essential throughout the year below 400m.
B. Subtropical humidity decreased by sea breezes. Rain frequent and heavy September—October.

Benin (People's Republic)
A.   Yellow fever — for those arriving within 6 days after leaving or transiting* infected areas (children under one year exempt).
Malaria prophylaxis essential throughout the country throughout the year. Chloroquine resistance reported.
B.   Tropical.   In   the   north   considerable   variation.   Rainy season July—October. Equatorial in south with two rainy seasons March—mid July and mid September—November. High humidity all the year.

Bermuda
A.   No vaccination demanded from any country.
B.   Semi-tropical, but cold winds prevail January to March. Hottest months August, September.

Bhutan
A.   Yellow fever — for all passengers including infants if arriving within 6 days after leaving or transiting* infected areas or endemic areas or Trinidad & Tobago.
Persons without valid yellow fever certificate, if required, are subject to quarantine for up to 6 days at their expense.
Malaria prophylaxis essential below 1600m throughout the year. Chloroquine and pyrimethamine/sulphadoxine resistance reported.
Climate varies according to altitude: in the south hot and humid, in summer, cold in winter in the mountainous north.

Bolivia
A.   Yellow fever — if arriving within 6 days after leaving or transiting* infected areas. All passengers going to Santa Cruz de la Sierra must be in possession of a valid yellow fever certificate but it is recommended for all passengers to Bolivia.
Malaria prophylaxis is essential throughout the year below 2,500m for all rural areas. Resistance to chloroquine reported.
B.   Entirely dependent on altitude. Can be tropical, temperate or cold. December—January rain practically daily. La Paz average 50°F.

Botswana
A.   Nil demanded from any country.
Malaria prophylaxis essential November through June in the northern part of the country (north of 21°S).
B.   Subtropical. Low humidity. Rainy season October— April.

Brazil
A. Yellow fever — if arriving within 6 days after leaving or transiting* infected areas. Recommended for all passengers visiting any area outside the main cities of Brazil. (Children under 6 months exempt). Malaria prophylaxis is essential throughout the year below 900m in Acre State, Territory of Amapa, Rondonia, Roraima, and in parts of rural areas of Amazonas, Goias, Maranhao, Mato Grosso and Para States. Chloroquine and sulphadoxine/pyrimethamine resistance reported.
B. Tropical. Very hot and humid. Heavy rainfall throughout.

British Virgin Islands
A. Nil demanded from any country.
B. Subtropical. Rainy season August—November. Constant tradewinds keep humidity down.

Brunei
A. Yellow fever — if arriving within 6 days after leaving or transiting* infected areas (children under one year exempt).
B. Tropical. Very hot and humid. Rain throughout the year. Wettest October—March.

Bulgaria
A. Nil demanded from any country.
B. Hot and dry in summer. Cold in winter.

Burkina Faso (formerly Upper Volta)
A. Yellow fever — (children under one year exempt).
Malaria prophylaxis essential throughout the country throughout the year. Chloroquine resistance reported.
B. Northern area hot and dry. Southern area hot and very humid. Rainy season July—October. Violent storms in August.

Burma (now Myanmar)
A. Yellow fever — if arriving within 6 days after leaving or transiting* infected areas or endemic area or leaving for a destination in an infected area (children under one year exempt).
Malaria prophylaxis essential thorughout the year in Karen State. From March through December elsewhere, except in Rangoon City. Chloroquine and sulphadoxine/pyrimethamine resistance is reported.
B. Tropical. Hot February—May. Monsoon May—October. Warm November—January. Rainfall may be over 20 inches per month in June, July and August. Humidity is always high.

Burundi

A. Yellow fever — if arriving within 6 days after leaving or transiting* infected areas (children under one year exempt). Recommended for all passengers visiting any areas outside the main cities in Burundi.
Malaria prophylaxis is essential throughout the year throughout the country. Chloroquine resistance reported.
B. Tropical. Hot and moderate humidity. Rainfall heavy February—May and December.

Cameroon

A. Yellow fever — (children under one year exempt).
Malaria prophylaxis is essential throughout the country throughout the year. Chloroquine resistance reported.
B. Tropical. Hot. Very humid on the coast: less so on the plateau. Dry November—May. Wet June—October.

Canada

A. Nil demanded from any country.
Immigrants have to be medically examined by appointed doctors before being granted immigrant visas. Any visitor, irrespective of length of intended stay in Canada, may be referred for medical examination if deemed necessary.
B. Complete variation according to time of year and location, from hot to very cold.

Canary Islands

A. Nil demanded.
B. Generally moderately warm and dry.

Cape Verde Islands

A. Nil demanded from any country.
Yellow fever — if arriving within 6 days after leaving or transiting* infected areas. Not required for entering Sao Vicente, Sal, Maio and Boa Vista (children under one year exempt).
Malaria prophylaxis essential throughout the year in rural areas.
B. Generally moderately warm and dry.

Cayman Islands

A. Nil demanded.
B. Subtropical to tropical. Torrential showers. Humidity fairly high. Hot season May—October.

Central African Republic
A.   Yellow fever — children under one year exempt. Required also for transit passengers not leaving the airport.
Malaria prophylaxis essential throughout the year throughout the country. Chloroquine resistance reported.
B.   Hot and humid. Rainy season June—October.

Chad
A.   Yellow fever — recommended for all passengers over one year.
Malaria prophylaxis is essential throughout the country throughout the year.
B.   Tropical. Very hot in northern district.

Chile
A.   Nil demanded from any country.
B.   Tropical in the north. Very cold in the South. Rainy season May—August. Santiago and Valparaiso Mediterranean.

China (People's Republic)
A.   Required *also* for transit passengers not leaving the airport:
Yellow fever — if arriving within 6 days after leaving or transiting* infected areas.
Malaria prophylaxis essential throughout the year throughout the country below 1,500m. Resistance to chloroquine reported.
B.   Climate can vary from one extreme to the other.

Christmas Island
A.   Yellow fever — if arriving from infected areas (children under one year exempt).
B.   Tropical. Dry May—September. Wet October—April.

Colombia
A.   Yellow fever — recommended for all passengers visiting any area outside the main cities in Colombia.
Malaria prophylaxis essential throughout the year in rural areas below 800m. Chloroquine and sulphadoxine/pyrimethamine resistance reported.
B.   Tropical, but temperature varies according to altitude but little variation throughout the year. Driest months December—February.

Comores Islands
A.   No vaccinations required.
Malaria prophylaxis essential throughout the year throughout the

Islands. Chloroquine resistance reported.
B. Tropical. Very humid and rainy October—March.

Congo (People's Republic)
A. Yellow fever — exempt are children under one year.
Malaria prophylaxis essential throughout the year throughout the country. Chloroquine resistance reported.
B. Tropical. Hot and humid. Dry season June—September.

Cook Islands
A. Nil demanded from any country.
B. Tropical. Wet December—March. Dry April—November.

Costa Rica
A. Nil demanded from any country.
Malaria prophylaxis is essential throughout the year in all rural areas below 500m.
B. Subtropical. Little variation throughout the year. Rainy season June—November.

Côte d'Ivoire
A. Yellow fever — children under one year exempt. Malaria prophylaxis essential throughout the country throughout the year.
B. Tropical. Hot and very humid at coast. Drier in north. Rainy season May—July, October—November.

Cuba
A. No vaccinations required from any country.
B. Subtropical. Rainy season May—October. Hurricanes August-October.

Cyprus
A. Nil demanded from any country.
B. Mediterranean. Summers hot and dry but increased humidity at the coast. Rainy season December—January.

Czechoslovakia
A. Nil demanded from any country.
B. Warm summers. Cold winters.

Denmark
A. Nil demanded from any country.
B. Temperate. Winters longer and colder than U.K.

Djibouti (Republic)
A. Yellow fever — if arriving within 6 days after leaving or transiting* infected areas — (children under one year exempt).
Malaria prophylaxis essential throughout the year throughout the country.
B. Hot and humid. May and September very hot. November—March relatively cool but heaviest rainfall.

Dominica
A Yellow Fever — if arriving within 6 days after leaving or transiting* infected areas — (children under one year exempt).
B Subtropical. Sunny but some wind. Rain May—November.

Dominican Republic
A. Nil demanded from any country.
Malaria prophylaxis essential throughout the year in rural areas.
B. Tropical. Little variation in the year. Dry season November—April.

Ecuador
A. Nil demanded but yellow fever strongly recommended for anyone visiting an area outside the main cities.
Malaria prophylaxis essential throughout the year below 1,500m. Chloroquine resistance reported.
B. Tropical on coast. Temperate in mountains. Subtropical foothills.

Egypt (Arab Republic of)
A.Yellow fever — if arriving within 6 days after leaving or transiting* infected areas, including any part of one of the following countries, (children under one year exempt).
Africa: Benin, Botswana, Burkina Faso, Burundi, Cameroon, Central African Republic, Chad, Congo, Côte d'Ivoire, Equatorial Guinea, Ethiopia, Gabon, Gambia, Ghana, Guinea, Guinea-Bissau, Kenya, Liberia, Malawi, Mali, Niger, Nigeria, Rwanda, Senegal, Sierra Leone, Somalia, Sudan (south of 15°N), Tanzania, Togo, Uganda, Zaire.
America: Belize, Bolivia, Brazil, Colombia, Costa Rica, Ecuador, French Guiana, Guatemala, Guyana, Honduras, Nicaragua, Panama, Peru, Surinam, Trinidad & Tobago, Venezuela.
Persons without valid yellow fever certificate, if required, are subject to quarantine.

Malaria prophylaxis essential from June through October in the Nile Delta, El Faiyum area, the oases, and Upper Egypt.
Cholera, Typhoid and Meningitis required if arriving from the Sudan. Diphtheria, Whooping Cough, Tetanus and Poliomyelitis required for children arriving from the Sudan.
B.   Cool and dry winters. Hot and fairly dry summers. Khamsin and dust storms April—May.

El Salvador
A.   Yellow fever — if arriving within 6 days after leaving or transiting* infected areas (children under 6 months exempt).
Malaria prophylaxis essential throughout the year throughout the country.
B.   Tropical — humid. Temperate in mountains. San Salvador is at 700m. Wet May—October.

Equatorial Guinea
A.   Yellow fever — if arriving within 6 days after leaving or transiting* infected areas. Recommended for everyone visiting any area outside the main cities.
Cholera and yellow fever vaccinations are recommended for everyone entering the country. Malaria prophylaxis essential throughout the year throughout the country.
B.   Tropical. Wet and humid. Rainy season May—September.

Ethiopia
A.   Yellow fever — (children under one year exempt).
Malaria prophylaxis essential throughout the year throughout the country below 2,000m. Chloroquine resistance reported.
B.   Lowlands hot and humid. Hill country warm and pleasant. Central uplands cool. Rainy season mid June—September and February—March.

Fiji
A.   Yellow fever — if arriving by air within 6 days after leaving or transiting* infected areas (children under one year exempt).
B.   Tropical. Very humid in Suva. Drier on Nadi coast. Monsoon November to May.

Finland
A.   Nil demanded from any country.
B.   Summer mild. Winter very cold.

France
A.   Nil demanded from any country.
B.   Temperate in the north to Mediterranean in the south.

French Guiana
A.   Yellow fever — for all passengers (children exempt under one year)
Malaria prophylaxis essential throughout the country throughout the year. Chloroquine resistance reported.
B.   Tropical. Hot and humid. Rainy season December—July.

French Polynesia
A.   Yellow fever — if arriving by air within 6 days after leaving or transiting* infected areas (children under one year exempt).
B.   Subtropical. Little variation. Occasional storms. Warmest and wettest in December—February.

French West Indies
A.   Yellow fever — if arriving within 6 days after leaving or transiting* infected areas (children under one year exempt).
B.   Subtropical. Sunny but some wind. Rain May—November.

Gabon
A.   Yellow fever — (children under one year exempt).
Malaria prophylaxis essential throughout the year throughout the country. Chloroquine resistance reported.
B.   Tropical. Hot and humid. Rainy seasons October—mid December and mid January—mid May.

Gambia
A.   Yellow fever — (children under one year exempt).
Malaria prophylaxis essential throughout the year throughout the country. Chloroquine resistance reported.
B.   Tropical. In general hot and humid. Rain June—October.

Germany, Federal Republic
A.   Nil demanded from any country.
B.   Temperate. Warm summers. Fairly cold winters.

Ghana
A. Yellow fever — (children under one year exempt).
Cholera recommended as a justifiable additional personal protection.
Malaria prophylaxis essential throughout the country throughout the year. Chloroquine resistance reported.
B. Tropical. Hot and humid except in the north, where it is dry. Rainy seasons April—July and September—October. Harmattan dry and dusty. North-east wind January — February.

Gibraltar
A. Nil demanded.
B. Temperate. Warm summers. Cool winters. Rainy seasons September—May.

Greece
A. Yellow fever — if arriving within 6 days after leaving or transiting* infected areas (children under 6 months exempt). Persons without a valid certificate, if required, are liable to quarantine.
B. Mediterranean, but cold in winter in north. In south in summer the temperature may rise to 110°F (43°C). Rain November—March.

Grenada
A. Yellow fever if arriving 6 days after leaving or transiting* infected areas.
B. Subtropical to tropical with high humidity. Wet season June—December.

Guam (Mariana Islands, U.S.A.)
A. See U.S.A.
B. Tropical. Hot and humid.

Guatemala
A. Yellow fever — if arriving within 6 days after leaving or transiting* infected areas (children under one year exempt).
Malaria prophylaxis essential throughout the year in rural areas below 1500m.
B. Coastal hot and humid. Mountains cool and dry.

Guinea-Bissau
A. Yellow fever — for those arriving within 6 days after leaving or transiting* infected areas and from the following countries:

Africa: Angola, Benin, Burkina Faso, Burundi, Central African Republic, Chad, Congo, Côte d'Ivoire, Djibouti, Equatorial Guinea, Ethiopia, Gabon, Gambia, Ghana, Guinea, Kenya, Liberia, Madagascar, Mali, Mauritania, Mozambique, Niger, Nigeria, Rwanda, São Tomé and Principe, Senegal, Sierra Leone, Somalia, Tanzania, Togo, Uganda, Zaire, Zambia.

America: Bolivia, Brazil, Colombia, Ecuador, French Guiana, Guyana, Panama, Peru, Surinam, Venezuela.

It is also recommended for all passengers visiting any area outside the main cities of Guinea (children under one year exempt).

Malaria prophylaxis essential throughout the country throughout the year.

B.   Tropical. Hot and humid. Marked wet and dry season. Rainy season mid May—mid November. Dry season mid November—mid May.

Guinea (Republic of)

A.   Yellow fever — except travellers from a non-infected area and children under one year, but recommended for all travellers visiting any area outside the main cities of Guinea.

Malaria prophylaxis essential throughout the year throughout the whole country.

B.   Tropical. Hot and humid. Drier in north. Wet season early May—late October. Dry November—April.

Guyana

A.   Yellow fever — if arriving within 6 days after leaving or transiting* infected areas and from:

Africa: Angola, Benin, Burkina Faso, Burundi, Cameroon, Central African Republic, Chad, Congo, Côte d'Ivoire, Ethiopia, Gabon, Gambia, Ghana, Guinea, Guinea-Bissau, Kenya, Liberia, Mali, Niger, Nigeria, Rwanda, São Tomé and Principe, Senegal, Sierra Leone, Somalia, Tanzania, Togo, Uganda, Zaire.

America: Belize, Bolivia, Brazil, Colombia, Costa Rica, Ecuador, French Guiana, Guatemala, Honduras, Nicaragua, Panama, Peru, Surinam, Venezuela.

But recommended for all passengers visiting any area outside the main cities of Guyana. Persons without valid yellow fever certificates, if required, will not be allowed to disembark.

Malaria prophylaxis essential throughout the year in the north-west region and in the Rupununi region. Chloroquine resistance reported.

B. Tropical. Hot and humid. Two wet seasons May—August and November—January.

Haiti
A. Yellow fever — if arriving within 6 days after leaving or transiting* infected areas.
Malaria prophylaxis essential throughout the year in all suburban and rural areas.
B. Subtropical. Cooler in mountains. Spring rains May and June. Main rains October and November.

Honduras
A. Yellow fever — if arriving within 6 days after leaving or transiting* infected areas.
Malaria prophylaxis essential throughout the year throughout the country.
B. Tropical. Hot and humid on coast. Cooler in mountains. Rains throughout year. Heavy September—February, particularly December and January.

Hong Kong
A. Nil demanded from any country.
B. Subtropical. Summers hot and humid. Winters sunny and dry. Cyclones July—September.

Hungary
A. Nil demanded from any country.
B. Summers very warm. Winters very cold. Little rain in summer.

Iceland
A. Nil demanded from any country.
B. Temperate with cool summers. Strong winds and gales in winter.

India
A. Cholera — if proceeding to countries imposing quarantine restrictions for arrivals from India or from an infected area in India. Vaccination against cholera could be considered as a justified additional personal protection.
Yellow fever — for all passengers including infants if arriving within 6 days after leaving or transiting* infected areas or any part of one of the following countries:

Africa: Angola, Benin, Botswana, Burkina Faso, Burundi, Cameroon, Central African Republic, Chad, Congo, Côte d'Ivoire, Equatorial Guinea, Ethiopia, Gabon, Gambia, Ghana, Guinea, Guinea-Bissau, Kenya, Liberia, Mali, Mauritania, Niger, Nigeria, Rwanda, São Tomé and Principe, Senegal, Sierra Leone, Somalia, Sudan (south of 15°N), Tanzania, Togo, Uganda, Zaire, Zambia.

America: Belize, Bolivia, Brazil, Colombia, Costa Rica, Ecuador, French Guiana, Guatemala, Guyana, Honduras, Nicaragua, Panama, Peru, Surinam, Trinidad & Tobago, Venezuela.

N.B. Vaccination is required for all persons even if only transiting the areas mentioned above. Persons without valid yellow fever certificate, if required, are subject to quarantine for a maximum 6 days.

Malaria prophylaxis essential throughout the year except the big cities. Chloroquine resistance reported.

B. Considerable variation. Very hot immediately previous to monsoon. Monsoon in Delhi, Bombay and Calcutta June—September. Madras heaviest October—November.

Indonesia

A. Yellow fever — if arriving within 6 days after leaving or transiting* infected areas or countries situated in endemic areas.

Cholera — strongly recommended.

Malaria prophylaxis is essential throughout the year throughout the country. Chloroquine and sulphadoxine/pyrimethamine resistance reported.

B. Tropical. Dry May—September. Wet October—April, worst January and February.

Iran (Islamic Republic of)

A. Yellow fever if arriving within 6 days after leaving or transiting* infected area (children under one year exempt).

NB Persons without valid certificates for yellow fever, if required, are subject to quarantine.

Malaria prophylaxis is essential from March through November below 1,500m except in Teheran and Shiraz. Chloroquine resistance reported.

B. High plateau — warm spring, hot summer, cold winter. Coast areas hot and humid. Dust storms July and August.

Iraq

A. Yellow fever — if arriving within 6 days after leaving or transiting* infected areas.

Malaria prophylaxis is essential from May through November in all areas below 1,500m.

Warning: All passengers arriving in Iraq intending to stay in Iraq more than 5 days must report for an AIDS test at Al Kindi, Al Kerama or El Kadhimiya hospital in Baghdad or one of the centres for preventive medicine outside Baghdad. Exempt from this are holders of an AIDS test certificate issued by a competent authority in Europe plus Canada, China, Japan and U.S.A. provided it is legalised by an Iraqi consulate.

B.   Summers extremely hot and dry, except Basra which is humid. Winters cool to cold.

Ireland (Republic)
A.   Nil demanded from any country.
B.   As in U.K. but slightly milder.

Israel
A.   Nil demanded from any country.
B.   Mediterranean. Humidity fairly high in summer. Rain November—March.

Italy
A.   Nil demanded from any country.
B.   Mediterranean. Winters can be cold in the north. Humid July—August.

Jamaica
A.   Yellow fever — if arriving within 6 days after leaving or transiting* infected areas (children under one year exempt).
B.   Tropical and humid at coast. Subtropical and humid inland. Cool at night December—March.

Japan
A.   Nil demanded from any country.
B.   Very cold in the north in the winter. Subtropical in the south in the summer. Hot and humid July and August. June rainy.

Jordan
A.   Nil demanded from any country.
B.   Extremely hot in valleys of River Jordan. Cooler in hills. Arid. All rainfall between November and March.

Kampuchea
A.   No reliable information can be obtained for Kampuchea.
B.   Tropical. Typical monsoon climate, hot and dry November–May. Heavy rain June—October. Humidity very high. Average temperature Phnom Penh 27°C (81°F) with minimal day and night variations.

Kenya
A.   Yellow fever — if arriving in Kenya from abroad within 6 days after leaving or transiting* endemic or infected areas outside Kenya. But strongly recommended for all passengers visiting any area outside the main cities in Kenya (children under one year exempt). Persons without valid yellow fever certificate, if required, are subject to quarantine.
Cholera — if arriving within 6 days after leaving or transiting* infected areas. (Children under one year exempt).
Typhoid vaccination strongly recommended by the authorities for all passengers entering Kenya.
Yellow fever vaccination recommended if visiting areas outside main cities (Children under one year exempt). Malaria prophylaxis essential throughout the year throughout the country. However, little risk above 2,500m. Chloroquine and sulphadoxine/pyrimethamine resistance reported.
B.   Hot and humid at coast. Hot and dry in the northern territories. Pleasantly warm in the highlands.

Kiribati (formerly Gilbert Islands)
A.   Yellow fever — if arriving within 6 days after leaving or transiting* infected areas (children under one year exempt). Also required for transit passengers not leaving the airport.
B.   Hot. Humid and rainy December through March.

Korea, Democratic People's Rep. of (North Korea)
A.   Nil demanded from any country.
B.   Winters dry and cold. Summers fairly hot. Humid July and August.

Korea, Republic of (South Korea)
A.   Nil demanded from any country.
B.   Winters dry and cold. Summers fairly hot. Humid July and August.

Kuwait
A. Nil demanded from any country.
B. Tropical. Extremely hot in summer. Humid in August. Winters comparatively cool. Rain November—January.

Laos
A. Yellow fever — if arriving within 6 days after leaving or transiting* infected areas.
Malaria prophylaxis essential throughout the year throughout the country. Chloroquine resistance reported.
B. Subtropical with great variations. South-west monsoon May to October.

Lebanon
A. Yellow fever — if arriving within 6 days after leaving or transiting* infected areas.
B. Mediterranean. Warm winters. Hot summers. Humid at coast. Snow in the mountains. Rain November—February.

Leeward Islands
Information applicable to British Virgin Islands and Anguilla, excluding Antigua and Barbuda (independent), Nevis, St Christopher (St Kitts), and Montserrat. (See separate entries under Antigua, and Netherlands Antilles.)
A. British Virgin Islands: Nil demanded from any country.
Anguilla and Montserrat: Yellow fever — if arriving within 6 days after leaving or transiting* infected area (children under one year exempt).
B. Sub tropical. Sunny but some wind. Rain August—November.

Lesotho
A. Yellow fever — if arriving within 6 days after leaving or transiting* infected areas. Also required for transit passengers not leaving the airport.
B. Hot and dry. Rainy season October—March.

Liberia
A. Yellow fever — children under one year exempt. Malaria prophylaxis throughout the year throughout the country.
B. Tropical. Hot and humid. Rainy season May—October.

Libya (Socialist People's Libyan Arab Jamahiriya)
A. Yellow fever — if arriving within 6 days after leaving or

transiting* infected areas. Children under one year exempt.
NB   For nationals of Libya and returning alien residents, health
certificates must have text translation printed in the Arab language.
Malaria prophylaxis is essential only in two small foci in the south
west of the country from February through August.
B.   Mediterranean on coast. Hot, dry and arid inland.

Luxembourg
A.   Nil demanded from any country.
B.   Temperate. Cool summers, mild winters. Rain fairly frequent.

Macao
A.   Nil demanded from any country.
B.   Subtropical. Summer hot and humid. Winter sunny and dry.
Wettest months April—September.

Madagascar (Democratic Republic of)
A.   Cholera if arriving within 6 days after leaving or transiting*
infected areas (children under one year exempt).
Yellow fever — if arriving within 6 days after leaving or transiting*
infected areas (children under one year exempt).
Malaria prophylaxis essential throughout the year throughout the
country. Chloroquine resistance reported.
B.   Tropical. April—October dry and warm at coast. Cold in the
highlands. November—March very hot on the coast, hot inland.

Malawi
A.   Yellow fever — if arriving within 6 days after leaving or
transiting* infected areas (children under one year exempt).
NB   Required for all passengers even if not leaving the airport in
Malawi.
Malaria prophylaxis essential throughout the year throughout the
country. High chloroquine and sulphadoxine/pyrimethine resistance
reported.
B.   Tropical, but wide variation according to altitude. Heavy rain
showers December—March.

Malaysia
The Federation of Malaysia includes Malaya and the Borneo states
of Sarawak and Sabah.
A.   Yellow fever — if arriving within 6 days after leaving or
transiting* countries with infected areas or countries with endemic
areas (children under one year exempt).

Malaria risk exists only in limited foci in the deep hinterland. Urban and coastal areas are free of malaria except in Sabah where there is risk throughout the year. High resistance to chloroquine and sulphadoxine/pyrimethamine reported.
B.   Tropical. Hot and humid. Little variation in the year. Wettest months October—March.

Maldive Islands
A.   Yellow fever — if arriving within 6 days after leaving or transiting* infected areas.
NB   Those not holding a valid yellow fever certificate, if required, will be vaccinated upon arrival and kept in quarantine at own expense for 10 days or otherwise deported by same flight.
Malaria prophylaxis essential throughout the year throughout the islands.
B.   Tropical with high humidity. March—May hot and dry. May—October SW monsoon, rain, winds and high seas. November—April north east monsoon dry and mild winds.

Mali
A.   Yellow fever — children under one year exempt
Malaria prophylaxis essential throughout the year throughout the country.
B.   Tropical. Hot and humid in south. Hot and dry in north. Rain July—September.

Malta
A.   Yellow fever — if arriving within 6 days after leaving infected areas. (Children under 6 months are exempt but are subject to isolation or surveillance when indicated).
B.   Mediterranean. Hot in summer. Cool in winter. Humid August, September.

Mauritania
A.   Yellow fever — if arriving within 6 days after leaving or transiting* infected areas and all passengers staying in Mauritania for longer than 2 weeks. But recommended for all other passengers visiting any area outside the main cities of Mauritania (children under one year exempt).
Malaria prophylaxis essential throughout the year throughout the country.
B.   Tropical. Warm and dry in the north. At coast warm October—May, hot and humid June—November.

Mauritius
A.   Yellow fever — if arriving within 10 days after leaving or transiting* infected areas and endemic areas (children under one year exempt).
Malaria prophylaxis essential throughout the year in rural areas in the north.
B.   Tropical maritime but no extremes. Humid at coast. Cold winds from the south and cyclones November—April.

Mayotte
A.   Yellow fever — if arriving within 6 days after leaving or transiting* infected areas (children under one year exempt).
B.   Tropical. Cooler in the inland hills. Cyclones December—March.

Mexico
A.   Yellow fever — if arriving within 6 days after leaving or transiting* infected areas (children under 6 months exempt).
Malaria prophylaxis is essential throughout the year throughout the rural and coastal areas.
B.   Varies to extremes with altitudes. Mexico City rainfall June—September.

Mongolia, People's Republic
A.   No reliable information can be obtained from Mongolia but last information was nil demanded.
B.   Extreme continental. Very cold in January: in north down to −34°C (−29°F), in south −19°C (−3°F). In July 15°C (59°F) and 23°C (74°F) respectively. But the rigours of the climate are to be a certain degree compensated by many days of sunshine (220—260 per year). The average elevation of the country is 1200m.

Montserrat and St Kitts-Nevis
A.   Yellow fever — if arriving within 6 days after leaving or transiting* countries with infected areas (children under one year exempt).
B.   Subtropical. Sunny but some wind. Rain August—November.

Morocco, including Tanger
A.   Nil demanded from any country.
Malaria prophylaxis strongly recommended from May through October in the rural areas.

B. Mediterranean in coastal areas. Hot and arid inland. Some rain November—March.

Mozambique
A. Yellow fever — if arriving within 6 days after leaving or transiting* infected areas (children under one year exempt).
Malaria prophylaxis essential throughout the year throughout the country. High chloroquine resistance reported.
B. Tropical. Warm and dry April—September. Hot, wet and very humid October—March.

Myanmar (see Burma)

Namibia
A. Yellow fever — if arriving within 6 days after leaving or transiting* infected or endemic areas. Persons without yellow fever certificate (if required) will be quarantined for 6 days or deported.
Malaria prophylaxis essential in northern swamp areas November—June. Chloroquine resistance reported.
B. Hot and dry on veld. Hot and humid at coast.

Nauru
A. Yellow fever — if arriving within 6 days after leaving or transiting infected areas. (NB Also for passengers not leaving the airport in Nauru.) Children under one year exempt.
B. Tropical. Hot and humid. Wettest December—March.

Nepal
A. Yellow fever — if arriving within 6 days after leaving or transiting* infected areas.
Malaria prophylaxis essential throughout the year in rural areas. Resistance to chloroquine reported.
B. Varies greatly — altitude and monsoon.

Netherlands
A. Nil demanded from any country.
B. Cool summers and moderate winters.

Netherlands Antilles
A. Yellow fever — if arriving within 6 days after leaving or transiting* infected areas (children under 6 months exempt).
B. Sunny and pleasant all the year with low humidity. Rain November—December.

New Caledonia
A. Yellow fever — if arriving within 6 days after leaving or transiting* infected or endemic areas (children under one year exempt).
The authorities recommend vaccination against typhoid fever.
B. Tropical, but cooled by trade winds. December—March warm but humid with moderate rainfall. April to November cool and dry. Known as the islands of Eternal Spring.

New Zealand
A. Nil demanded from any country.
B. Great variation between north and south. Summers generally dry. Snow in winter in south.

Nicaragua
A. Yellow fever — for those arriving within 6 days after leaving or transiting* infected areas (children under one year exempt).
Malaria prophylaxis essential throughout the year in all rural areas below 1,000m (and outskirts of towns).
B. Tropical. Hot throughout the year. Dry November—May. Wet and humid May—November.

Niger
A. Yellow fever — children under one year exempt.
Malaria prophylaxis essential throughout the year throughout the country.
B. Tropical. Hot and dry. Heaviest rain in August. November—January cooler when the Harmattan blows off the desert.

Nigeria
A. Yellow fever — children under one year exempt.
Malaria prophylaxis essential throughout the year throughout the country. Chloroquine resistance reported.
B. Hot. Humid in the south. Dry in the north. Rainy season in south March—November; in north April—September.

Niue
A. Yellow fever — for those arriving within 6 days after leaving or transiting* infected areas (children under one year exempt).
B. Tropical. Wet December—March. Dry April—November.

Norfolk Island
A. Nil demanded from any country.
B. Subtropical. Hot and humid. Coolest months June—August.

Northern Mariana Islands (Micronesia)
A. Nil demanded from any country.
B. Hot and humid. Wettest period May—November; within the typhoon belt.

Norway
A. Nil demanded from any country.
B. Summers cool. Winters cold. Snowfall November—March.

Oman
A. Yellow fever — if arriving within 6 days after leaving or transiting* infected areas.
Cholera — travellers arriving with the intention of taking up residence will be subject to preventive measures against cholera prescribed by the Health Administration.
B. Very hot and humid in summer, May—October. Worst months July—September. Very pleasantly mild December—March.

Pakistan
A. Cholera — if arriving within 5 days after leaving or transiting* infected areas.
Yellow fever — if arriving within 6 days after leaving or transiting* infected or endemic areas. (NB Persons without a valid yellow fever certificate, if required, are subject to quarantine.)
Exempt are infants under 6 months if the mother's vaccination certificate shows that she has been duly vaccinated prior to the birth of the baby.
Malaria prophylaxis essential throughout the year throughout the country below 2,000m. Resistance to chloroquine reported.
B. Very hot and generally dry in summer. Monsoon usually July—September with high humidity. Usually fine and dry November—March but freezing in the north-west.

Panama
A. Yellow fever — for all travellers visiting any areas out side the main cities of Panama.
Malaria prophylaxis essential throughout the year throughout the rural areas. Chloroquine resistance reported.

B.   Tropical. Hot all the year, cooler inland. Very heavy rainfall October—November.

Papua New Guinea
A.   Yellow fever — if arriving within 6 days after leaving or transiting* infected areas (children under one year exempt). (NB Persons without valid vaccination certificates, if required, are subject to quarantine.)
Malaria prophylaxis essential throughout the year throughout the country. Chloroquine resistance reported.
B.   Tropical. Hot for most of the year. No recognised seasons. north-west monsoon December—March, wet. South-east tradewinds May—December, dry. Cool in highlands.

Paraguay
A.   Yellow fever — if arriving within 6 days after leaving or transiting* infected areas (children under 6 months exempt).
Malaria prophylaxis essential from October through May in rural areas.
B.   Sub tropical summer and warm. Rainiest season October—April but there can be heavy rain any time of the year.

Peru
A.   Yellow fever — if arriving within 12 days after leaving or transiting* infected areas; and recommended for all passengers visiting any area outside the main cities of Peru (children under 6 months exempt).
Malaria prophylaxis essential throughout the year in all rural areas below 1,500m. Chloroquine resistance reported.
B.   Varies from temperate to tropical according to region but generally humid or wet. Heaviest rainfall October—April. Coastal areas (Lima) very little sunshine due to cold sea mist.

Philippines
A.   Yellow fever — if arriving within 6 days after leaving or transiting* infected areas. Children under one year are exempt but are subject to isolation or surveillance when it is indicated.
Malaria prophylaxis is essential throughout the year in all rural areas below 600 metres. Chloroquine resistance reported.
A valid AIDS clearance certificate is required for those staying longer than 6 months.
B.   Tropical. Hot and always humid. Wet season July—October.

Hot, dusty and humid March—June. Relatively cool November—February.

Poland
A. Nil demanded from any country.
B. Temperate but summers tend to be very warm and winters cold. Rainfall comparatively high.

Portugal
A. Yellow fever — (for Azores and Madeira only) except for transit passengers staying not more than 4 days and not leaving landing Island, if arriving within 6 days after leaving or transiting* infected areas. Children under one year exempt.
B. Temperate in the north-west, moderate winters. Abundant rain, short summers. North-east: long cold winters, hot summers. South: moderate winters, long hot summers, very little rain.
Madeira: subtropical, slightly humid. Rain mainly November—March.
Azores: spring and autumn season short. Winter is damp and rainy with violent gales. July and August hot and humid. Early summer best.

Puerto Rico (U.S.A.)
A. For requirements see U.S.A.
B. Tropical maritime with little temperature variations. June—October tends to have more rain.

Qatar
A. Yellow fever — if arriving within 6 days after leaving or transiting* infected areas (children under one year exempt).
B. Exceptionally hot and humid in the summer. Mild in the winter.

Reunion
A. Yellow fever — if arriving after leaving or transiting* infected areas (children under one year exempt).
B. Tropical. St Denis on windward side hot and humid. St Pierre drier. Cooler in the inland hills. Cyclones December—March.

Romania
A. Nil demanded from any country.
B. Continental. Hot summers, long cold winters (November—March). Milder on Black Sea coast.

Rwanda
A. Yellow fever — children under one year exempt.
Malaria prophylaxis essential throughout the year throughout the country. High chloroquine resistance reported.
B. Tropical. Hot and humid but considerably cooler in mountains. Two rainy seasons in year. Long rains mid January—mid May. Short rains mid October—mid December.

Samoa (American)
A. Yellow fever — if arriving within 6 days after leaving or transiting* infected areas (children under one year exempt). (NB Also required for passengers not leaving the airport in Samoa.)
B. Tropical. Wet with heavy rainfall December—March. Dry with south-east tradewinds April—November. Cyclones and tropical storms can be a hazard.

Samoa (Western)
A. Yellow fever — if arriving within 6 days after leaving or transiting* infected areas (children under one year exempt). (NB Also required for passengers not leaving the airport in Samoa).
B. Tropical. Cooler months May—November. Rainy season December—April.

Sao Tomé and Principe
A. Yellow fever — if arriving within 6 days after leaving or transiting* infected areas and for all passengers staying in São Tomé and Principe for longer than 2 weeks; but recommended for all passengers visiting rural areas (children under one year exempt).
Malaria prophylaxis essential throughout the year throughout the country.
B. Equatorial with heavy rainfall, high temperatures and high humidity. Dry mid September—May. Wet June—mid September.

Saudi Arabia
A. Yellow fever — if arriving within 6 days after leaving or transiting* infected areas. (NB Persons without valid yellow fever certificates, if required, will be vaccinated upon arrival *and* are subject to quarantine.)
Malaria prophylaxis essential throughout the year other than in the main cities.
Meningitis. At time of Haj Pilgrimage and entering via Jeddah meningitis vaccination is required.

B. Desert. Red Sea coastal areas (Jeddah) hot and humid throughout the year. Interior (Riyadh) extremely hot in summer (up to 50°C/122°F) cold in winter. Occasional heavy rain November—February. Gulf coast hot and humid. Dust storms May—September in the east.

Senegal
A. Yellow fever — children under one year exempt.
(NB Passengers arriving without a valid yellow fever certificate will be refused entry.)
Malaria prophylaxis essential throughout the year throughout the country.
B. Tropical. Coastal areas hot and humid. Interior extremely hot and dry. Rainy season July—October.

Seychelles
A. Nil demanded from any country.
B. Equable with only slight variations. Coolest June—October with south-east trade winds. Hottest December—April with north-west monsoons.

Sierra Leone
A. Yellow fever recommended for all passengers visiting any area outside the main cities of Sierra Leone also for anyone arriving within 6 days after leaving or transiting* infected areas. Certificate may be required for those leaving.
Malaria prophylaxis essential throughout the year throughout the country.
B. Tropical and humid. Rainfall very heavy especially in Freetown and coastal areas (3300mm per year). Wet season mid May—mid November heaviest July—September. Harmattan dry wind from the Sahara December—January.

Singapore
A. Yellow fever — if arriving within 6 days after leaving or transiting* countries any parts of which are endemic or infected (children under one year exempt). (NB Persons without valid yellow fever certificate, if required, are subject to quarantine. May be sent back to the port of embarkation. Letters of exemption are not acceptable.)
B. Tropical. Hot and humid. Probably the least variable climate in the world. Heavy monsoons November—February.

Solomon Islands
A. Yellow fever — if arriving within 6 days after leaving or transiting* infected areas.
Malaria prophylaxis essential throughout the year throughout the islands. Chloroquine resistance reported.
B. Tropical. Hot and humid. Wet season November—April. Tropical storms may be severe.

Somalia
A. Yellow fever — if arriving within 6 days after leaving or transiting* infected areas. Recommended for all visitors. (NB Persons without valid yellow fever certificate, if required, are subject to quarantine.)
Malaria prophylaxis essential throughout the year throughout the country.
B. Tropical. Hot, dry and arid in north. Hot and fairly humid in south.

South Africa, Republic of
A. Yellow fever — if arriving within 6 days after leaving or transiting* infected areas or African countries situated in the endemic areas. (NB Required for transit passengers not leaving the airport in South Africa.) Babies under one year are exempt provided a medical certificate can be submitted stating it is undesirable to vaccinate the baby. Persons without yellow fever certificate, if required, will be quarantined for six days or deported to country of origin.
Malaria prophylaxis essential throughout the year in the north, east and western low altitude areas of the Transvaal and the Natal coastal areas north of 28°S (Richard's Bay). Chloroquine resistance reported.
B. Temperate to sub tropical. Veld hot and dry, cool winters. Natal and Transvaal hot and humid, warm winters. Cape Province Mediterranean but can be cold in winter. No continuous rainy season.

Spain
A. Nil demanded from any country.
B. Temperate in the north. Hot and dry in the south.

Sri Lanka, Republic of
A. Yellow fever — if arriving within 6 days after leaving or transiting* infected areas (children under one year exempt). (NB

Persons without valid yellow fever certificate, if required, are subject to quarantine.)

Malaria prophylaxis essential throughout the year throughout the country. High chloroquine resistance reported.

B. Tropical. Cool in hills. Two monsoon periods. April—September mainly in south-west. October—March in the north-east. Humid in coastal areas.

St Kitts-Nevis

A. Yellow fever — if arriving within 6 days after leaving or transiting* infected areas (children under one year exempt).

B. Subtropical, sunny but some wind. Rain August—November.

St Lucia, St Vincent and the Grenadines

A. Yellow fever — if arriving within 6 days after leaving or transiting* infected or endemic areas (children under one year exempt).

B. Tropical but tempered by trade winds. February—May driest. Rain July—September

Sudan

A. Yellow fever — if arriving within 6 days after leaving or transiting* infected or endemic areas. Children under one year exempt, but recommended for all passengers visiting any areas outside the main cities in the Sudan. (NB A certificate may be required from travellers leaving the Sudan.)

Malaria prophylaxis essential throughout the year throughout the country. Chloroquine resistance reported.

B. Tropical north rather than south. Mid April—late June extremely hot and dry. July—September with rain, temperature drops but humidity high. April—September sand storms (*haboobs*) blow across from the Sahara. Best months October—mid April.

Surinam

A. Yellow fever — if arriving within 6 days after leaving or transiting* infected areas; but recommended for all passengers visiting any area outside the main cities of Surinam. Babies under one year are allowed to travel without a yellow fever vaccination certificate, provided a medical certificate is submitted stating that it is undesirable to inoculate the baby.

Malaria prophylaxis essential throughout the year throughout the

country. Chloroquine resistance reported.
B. Tropical. High rainfall. High humidity — little variation throughout the year or in the 24 hours.

Swaziland
A. Yellow fever — if arriving within 6 days after leaving or transiting* infected areas, this includes passengers not leaving the airport. Babies under one year are exempt provided a medical certificate is submitted stating that it is undesirable to vaccinate the baby.
Malaria prophylaxis essential throughout the year in all lowveld areas. Chloroquine resistance is reported.
B. Generally warm. Can be very hot and humid in the low veld in the summer. No continuous rainy season.

Sweden
A. Nil demanded from any country.
B. Very cold in north. Summer in central districts may be rather warm, winter cold throughout.

Switzerland and Liechtenstein
A. Nil demanded from any country.
B. Varies greatly with altitude. Generally warm summers and cold winters.

Syria
A. Yellow fever — if arriving within 6 days after leaving or transiting* infected areas.
Malaria prophylaxis essential from May through October throughout the country except Damascus, Homs and Tartus.
B. Basically Mediterranean. Hot dry summers, fairly cold winters. Rainfall November—March only.

Tahiti
See French Polynesia.

Taiwan (Formosa)
A. Nil demanded from any country.
B. Subtropical, long sultry summers May—October. Rainy season — north October—March, south May—September. Rain can be heavy and prolonged. Lies in the typhoon track.

Tanzania, United Republic of

A. Cholera — only if visiting Zanzibar or Pemba.

Yellow fever — children under one year exempt.

Government authorities recommend vaccination against typhoid.

Malaria prophylaxis essential throughout the year throughout the country below 1,800m. High resistance to chloroquine and sulphadoxine/pyrimethamine reported.

B. Tropical but varies greatly with altitude. Coastal areas hot and humid. Rainy in March—May. Central plateau dry and arid. Northwestern highlands cool and temperate. Rain in November—December, February—May.

Thailand

A. Yellow fever — if arriving within 6 days after leaving or transiting* infected and endemic areas. Those not holding a valid yellow fever vaccination certificate, if required, will be vaccinated on arrival and kept in quarantine for 6 days or otherwise deported.

Malaria prophylaxis essential throughout the year in rural, especially forested and hilly, areas of the whole country. High resistance to chloroquine and resistance to sulphadoxine/pyrimethamine reported.

B. Tropical. Warm and temperate in the northern mountains. Hot and humid in the south, tropical monsoon climates. Rainy and hot May—October.

Togo

A. Yellow fever — for all passengers (children under one year exempt).

Malaria prophylaxis essential throughout the year throughout the country. Chloroquine resistance reported.

B. Hot and humid especially at coast. Rainy seasons April—July and October—November.

Tonga

A. Yellow fever — if arriving within 6 days after leaving or transiting* infected areas (children under one year exempt). (NB Required also for all transit passengers not leaving the airport.)

B. Fairly high humidity but slightly cooler than most tropical areas. Hot season December—January.

Trinidad and Tobago

A. Yellow fever — if arriving within 6 days after leaving or transiting* infected areas or countries any parts of which are infected. Recommended for anyone visiting any area outside the main cities of Trinidad and Tobago. Children under one year exempt.

B. Tropical heat of Trinidad is tempered by the trade winds. 'Dry' season January—May. 'Wet' season June—September. Wettest month June.

Tunisia
A. Yellow fever — if arriving within 6 days after leaving or transiting* infected areas (children under one year exempt).
Malaria prophylaxis is essential in rural and coastal areas May—November.
B. Hot summers and mild winters. Rain light but frequent December—March. In the interior summer temperature can exceed 45°C (113°F).

Turkey
A. Nil demanded from any country.
Malaria prophylaxis essential from March to November inclusive in rural and coastal areas.
B. Considerable variation. Hot dry summers except on the north coast. Snow especially in east December—March. Heaviest rainfall winter and spring.

Tuvalu Republic (formerly Ellice Islands)
A. Yellow fever — if arriving within 6 days after leaving or transiting* infected areas (children under one year exempt). Required also for transit passengers not leaving the airport.
B. Semi tropical with two marked seasons. March—October cool and dry. November—March westerly gales and rain, hot and humid.

Uganda
A. Yellow fever — for all passengers over one year.
Malaria prophylaxis essential throughout the year throughout the country. Chloroquine resistance reported.
B. Generally warm late December to end of March. Hot in lake areas with high humidity particularly before rains. Long rains April—June. Short rains October—November. Cool season July—September.

United Arab Emirates
A. Yellow fever — if arriving within 6 days after leaving or

transiting* infected areas.
Malaria prophylaxis is essential in the foothills and valleys in the mountainous area of the northern emirates. It is recommended elsewhere.
B. May—October extremely hot and humid, especially July—September. (Average temp. 44°C (111°F) and 85% humidity.) December—March very pleasant and mild.

United Kingdom
A. Nil demanded from any country.
B. Temperate maritime. Rainfall throughout year.

Uruguay
A. Nil demanded from any country.
B. Mediterranean type, extremes of temperature rare. Rainfall basically spread evenly throughout year but heaviest July—August.

U.S.A.
A. Nil demanded from any country.
B. Continental from Arctic (Alaska) to Tropic of Cancer (Hawaii).

U.S.S.R.
A. Nil demanded from any country.
B. Varies from subarctic to subtropical. European Russia, warm summers with long, cold winters. Heavy snowfall north and east of Moscow. Murmansk and Siberia, cool summers with very long hard winters. Black Sea area, hot summers and mild winters.

Vanuatu (formerly New Hebrides)
A. Nil demanded from any country.
Malaria prophylaxis essential throughout the year throughout the area, except Futura Island. Chloroquine and sulphadoxine/pyrimethamine resistance reported.
B. Tropical. Hot December—April when tropical storms and cyclones may be a hazard. Heavy rainfall and high humidity.

Venezuela
A. Nil demanded from any country.
Yellow fever — strongly recommended for everyone visiting outside the main cities of Venezuela.
Malaria prophylaxis essential throughout the year in rural areas. Resistance to chloroquine reported.

B. Tropical. Little seasonal change but great variation with altitude. Caracas maximum temperature 32°C (90°F) July—August. Maracaibo hot and very humid. Rainy season May—November.

Vietnam Socialist Republic
A. Yellow fever — if arriving within 6 days after leaving or transiting* infected areas (children under one year exempt).
Malaria prophylaxis essential throughout the year throughout the country except urban areas and the delta. High resistance to chloroquine reported.
B. Tropical in south. Hot and humid. Monsoon climate. May—October generally hot. November—April usually dry.

Virgin Islands (U.S.A.)
A. Requirements as for U.S.A.
B. Subtropical. Sunny but some wind. Rain August—November.

Yemen Arab Republic
A. Nil demanded from any country.
Yellow fever — if arriving within 6 days after leaving or transiting* infected areas (children under one year exempt). (NB Deportation in case of non-compliance.)
Malaria prophylaxis essential throughout the year throughout the country.
B. Extremely hot and humid in coastal areas. Cooler in the highlands. Rainfall usually July—September.

Yemen People's Democratic Republic
(previously Aden Town and Western & Eastern Aden Protectorate)
A. Yellow fever — if arriving within 6 days after leaving or transiting* infected areas, Djibouti Rep., Ethiopia, Kenya, Somalia (children under one year exempt). Non-compliance will result in vaccination on arrival.
Malaria prophylaxis essential throughout the year except in Aden Town.
B. June—September hot with high humidity. Winter months pleasantly warm and dry — average 28°C (82°F). Cooler and drier on the high plateau. Rain almost non-existent.

Yugoslavia
A. Nil demanded from any country.

B. Mediterranean on the coastal strip, mild winters and hot summers. Alpine in the mountains with heavy snowfalls in the winter. In the north cold winters and hot summers.

Zaire
A. Yellow fever — (children under one year exempt).
Typhoid and cholera strongly recommended by Government.
Malaria prophylaxis essential throughout the year throughout the country. Resistance to chloroquine reported.
B. Tropical. Central and western, hot and humid. East and south-eastern, cooler and drier. Rainy seasons, south west October—May, equatorial zone throughout the year, north September—October and April—June, south and south east October—April.

Zambia
A. Yellow fever — if arriving within 6 days after leaving or transiting* infected areas; vaccination recommended for all passengers visiting outside the main cities (children under one year exempt).
Malaria prophylaxis essential throughout the year throughout the country. High chloroquine resistance reported. Cholera recommended for all passengers.
B. Subtropical to temperate in the high plateau areas. Rainy season mainly November—April, heavier December—January.

Zimbabwe
A. Yellow fever — if arriving within 6 days after leaving or transiting* infected areas.
Malaria prophylaxis essential throughout the year in all areas below 1,500m.
B. Generally healthy and very pleasant. Hot seasons mid August—mid November. Rainy season mid November—mid March. Heaviest December—January.

Transit document check sheet

In the countries mentioned below the authorities require in certain cases every transit passenger proceeding by the same flight and not leaving the aircraft to hold a valid YELLOW FEVER CERTIFICATE.

Central African Rep. Malawi   South Africa

China People's Rep.	Nauru	Swaziland
Kiribati	Samoa (American)	Tonga
Lesotho	Samoa (Western)	Tuvalu

Bibliography

ADAM, J.M. (1955) *A general view of the physiological problems arising in the Army*. Report to the War Office AMD5.

ADAM, J.M. (1967) *Climate and clothing*. Practitioner 198.645.

ADAM, J.M., LATHAM, F., and WYATT, H.T. (1963) *Preliminary observations of the immediate effect of heat on acclimatised paratroops.*. APRC Report 61/31 MRC.

BULMER, E. (1944) Survey of tropical diseases seen in the Middle East. *Transactions of the Royal Society of Tropical Medicine and Hygiene* 37.3225.

CLARKE, C. (1987) *Acclimatization, Acute Mountain Sickness and Travel to High Altitude.* Expedition Medicine.

CLUVER, E.H. (1964) (Letter) *South African Medical Journal.* 1964.38.

DAVIES, C.N., DAVIS, P.R., and TYRER, F.H. (1967). *The effects of abnormal physical conditions at work*. E. & S. Livingstone Ltd., Edinburgh.

De KRUIF, Paul (1927) *Microbe hunters*. Jonathan Cape.

DOROLLE, P. (1968) Old plagues in the jet age. *B.M.J.* 1968.4.789.

'ENDEAVOUR' JOURNAL OF JOSEPH BANKS F.R.S. (1767—1771), THE. Edited by J.C. Beaglehole (1961)

ENGEL, Arnold (1968) *Health effects of sunlight exposure in the U.S.A.* First National Health and Nutrition Examination Survey.

GOLDSMITH, R. (1967) Temperature control and environment. *Practitioner* 198.651.

GORDON, J.E. (1965) *Control of communicable diseases in man.* American Public Health Association.

HAGGARD, Howard W. (1941) *Devils, drugs and doctors.* William Heinemann.

HANEVELD, D. (1960). Epidemiological aspects of traveller's diarrhoea in the Lebanon. *Tropical and Geographical Medicine* 1960.12.339.

HAUTY, G.T. and ADAMS, J. (1966). Phase shifts of the human circadian system and performance of deficit during the periods of transition. 1. East—West Flight. *Aerospace Medicine* V.37.7. 2. West—East Flight. *Aerospace Medicine* V.37.19. 3. North—South Flight. *Aerospace Medicine* V.37.12.

KEAN, B.H. and WATERS, S.R. (1958). Incidence of diarrhoea in travellers returning to U.S. from Mexico. *A.M.A. Archives of Industrial Health.* 1958.18.148.

KEAN, B.H. and WATERS, S.R. (1959). Drug prophylaxis in Mexico. *New England Journal of Medicine* 1959.261.71.

KEAN, B.H., SCHAFFNER, W., BRENNAN, R.W. and WATERS, S.R. (1962). Prophylaxis with phthalylsulpha-thiazole and neomycin. *Journal of the American Medical Association* 1962.5.367.

LEITHEAD, C.S. and LIND, A.R. (1964) *Heat stress and heat disorders.* Cassell.

MACKIE, R.M. and AITCHISON, T. (1982). Severe sunburn and subsequent risk of primary cutaneous malignant melanoma in Scotland.

MACKIE, R.M. (1987) Links between exposure to ultra violet radiation and skin cancer. A report of The Royal College of Physician.

MANSON-BAHR, Sir Philip (1966) *Mansons tropical diseases.*

McFARLAND, R.A. (1953). *Human factors in air transportation.* McGraw-Hill.

McGIRR, P.O.M. (1967). Circadian rhythms in flight. *Transactions of the Society of Occupational Medicine* 1967.18.3.

McGREGOR, I. (1946) (Letter) *British Medical Journal* 1946.225. Cassell.

O'ROURKE, M.G.E. and EMMETT, A.J.J. (1982). *Malignant skin tumours in Australia.* Churchill Livingstone.

OWEN, Raymond J. (1968) *Medical report on Olympic Games.* British Olympic Association.

PIEKARSKI, G. (1962) *Medical parasitology.* Farbenfabriken Bayer A.G.

POLLOCK, T.M. and REID, D. (1969) Immunoglobulin for the prevention of infectious hepatitis in persons working overseas. *Lancet* 1969.1.28.

REID, H.A. (1968) Snake bite in the tropics. *British Medical Journal* 1968.3.359.

ROWE, B., TAYLOR, Joan, and BETTELHEIM, K.A. (1970). An investigation of travellers diarrhoea. *Lancet* 1970.1.1.

SHEPHERD, R.D. and BARLOW, J. (1962). *The effects of travel fatigue and tropical conditions on the military efficiency of unacclimatised parachute troops during the first three days.* APRC Report 61/26 MRC.

STEFFEN, R. and GSELL, O. (1981) Prophylaxis of traveller's diarrhoea. *Journal of Tropical Medicine and Hygiene* 84.239.

TURNER, A.C. (1967) Travellers diarrhoea. Survey of symptoms, occurrence and possible prophylaxis. *British Medical Journal* 1967.4.653.

TURNER, A.C. (1968). Some medical aspects of air travel. *Bulletin of British Association of Sport and Medicine.*

TURNER, A.C. (1968) Athletes and air travel. *Coaching review of Canada.*

TURNER, A.C. (1970). Keeping fit in worldwide business and holiday travel. *Transactions of the Society of Occupational Medicine.*

TURNER, A.C. (1971) Food poisoning. *Practitioner* V. 206.615.

TURNER, A.C. (1975) *Travel Medicine. A handbook for practitioners.* Churchill Livingstone Ltd, London & Edinburgh.

TURNER, A.C. (1978) Immunization for overseas travel. *Practitioner* V. 220.

TURNER, A.C. (1979) Fever in the international traveller. *Medicine International.*

TURNER, A.C. (1982) Is this person fit to fly? *Medicine in practice.*

TURNER, A.C. (1982) Prevention of malaria. *International Management.*

TURNER A.C. (1989). Can flying cause problems? — Guide to Travellers health. *Pulse.*

TURNER, A.C. (1989). The Travel Bug. *Chemist and Pharmacist.* Update.

TURNER, A.C. (1989). Malaria in Britain. *Travel Medicine International.*

TURNER, A.C., BARNES, R.M., and GREEN, R.L. (1971) The effect of a preparation of Vitamin A and calcium carbonate on sunburn. *Practitioner.* V. 206.

VARELA, G., KEAN, B.H., BARRETT, E.L., and KEEGAN, C.J. (1959) Bacteriological studies of U.S. students in Mexico. *American Journal of Tropical Medicine and Hygiene* 1959.8.353.

WARRELL, A.W. and BELL, S. (1978). *Synopsis of infectious and tropical diseases.* Wright & Son.

WOODRUFF, A.W. and BELL, S. (1978) *Synopsis of infectious and tropical diseases.* Wright and Son.

WOODSON, R.D. and CLINTON J.J. (1969) *Journal of the American Medical Association* 209.1053.

D. of H. Leaflets S.A. 30 and 36.

W.H.O. *International Health Regulations*

W.H.O. *Weekly Epidemiological Review*

W.H.O. *Malaria and Yellow Fever Maps*

Index